Advance Praise for
A Funny Thing Happened on the Way to Stockholm

"Lefkowitz unveils the teamwork, persistence, and labors of love that go into living a life of significance. By turns funny and moving, this book has the power to inspire."

—**Mike Krzyzewski, Head Coach,**
Men's Basketball, Duke University

"An engaging Nobel Prize-winning journey of a life in medicine and science. Joyous, insightful, and irreverent, Lefkowitz describes the enormous impediments to challenging established dogma and legendary elders as well as the art and satisfaction of mentoring young scientists. For both lay readers and professional scientists this book presents a narrative that will delight and that offers a goldmine of wisdom."

—**Robert Horvitz, Ph.D., Massachusetts Institute of Technology,**
Investigator of the Howard Hughes Medical Institute;
Nobel Prize in Physiology or Medicine (2002)

"A tribute to teamwork that aims to inspire the young generation of scientists to take a similar journey. This book shows that making a breakthrough discovery, changing a paradigm, and using science as a tool to change people's lives is possible, while also emphasizing that such achievements are not made by angels but by human beings like all of us."

—**Aaron Ciechanover, M.D., D.Sc., Technion, Israel Institute**
of Technology, Nobel Prize in Chemistry (2004)

"Lefkowitz's life is testament to the joy of science. The book is a page-turner, a riveting account of a life well-lived. It is a story of stories, a tale of greatness."

—**Roger D. Kornberg, Ph.D., Stanford University,**
Nobel Prize in Chemistry (2006)

"Lefkowitz appreciates the power of storytelling, both at the bedside in making diagnoses and at the bench in generating hypotheses. Full of vignettes that are sometimes embarrassingly honest, at other times laugh-out-loud humorous, but always infused with his own special brew of humility and hubris. An informative and entertaining read."

—**Helen H. Hobbs, M.D., Investigator,**
Howard Hughes Medical Institute,
University of Texas Southwestern Medical Center

"In this engaging and often rollicking tale, Bob Lefkowitz recounts how the Vietnam War transformed him from a dedicated young physician into an enthusiastic, ambitious, and highly successful scientist whose discoveries have altered our understanding of cell function and approaches to drug development. Arriving at a time when the need to convert physicians into scientists is greater than ever, this book can do more than just entertain and instruct: it can inspire young doctors to remake their careers."

—**Harold Varmus, M.D., Lewis Thomas University Professor, Weill Cornell Medicine; Nobel Prize in Physiology or Medicine (1989); Author of** *The Art and Politics of Science*

"A master story-teller, Bob Lefkowitz shares his journey as one of our preeminent biomedical scientists. For any aspiring clinical or biomedical scholar, and their anxious parents, you will see how one of our country's most distinguished medical scholars navigated his life to the top."

—**Randy Schekman, Ph.D., University of California, Berkeley, Nobel Prize in Physiology or Medicine (2013)**

"In this entertaining book, Nobelist Bob Lefkowitz recounts how he became a passionate and renowned physician-scientist. He unveils the secret to his scientific stardom in a series of engrossing stories spanning his fifty-year career. No tale is left untold—many are amusing, some might raise a few eyebrows."

—**Joseph L. Goldstein, M.D., and Michael S. Brown, M.D., U.T. Southwestern Medical Center, Nobel Prizes in Physiology or Medicine (1985)**

"Lighthearted, yet profoundly personal and moving, Lefkowitz's memoir shares the secret recipe for winning a Nobel prize—two parts genius, one part audacity in challenging authority, one part insightful and supportive mentoring, a splash of good luck, and ten parts resilience and persistence. Bob Lefkowitz is at the top of the list of the extraordinary cadre of physicians turned scientists who ushered in the modern biotechnology revolution."

—**Barry S. Coller, M.D., David Rockefeller Professor of Medicine, Rockefeller University, Physician-in Chief, Rockefeller University Hospital**

"The odds of a scrappy kid growing up in the Bronx winning a Nobel Prize are overwhelmingly small. How Bob Lefkowitz managed to do this is revealed in this delightfully rich and moving book allowing the reader to understand Bob's intelligence, warmth, and complexity. If you read one book this year, choose this one. It will fill you with joy, hope, and give you a new friend."

—**Ralph Snyderman, M.D., Professor of Medicine, Chancellor Emeritus, Duke University**

"More than just a heartwarming and thrilling chronicle of a great physician-scientist, Lefkowitz has written a story-based leadership guide for any aspiring mentor. A testament to the power of building enduring excellence by believing in, championing, and developing others."

—**Sanyin Siang, Leadership Coach and author of** *The Launch Book*

"How does a brilliant young physician accidentally get hooked on research? Bob Lefkowitz's life-altering shift changed not only his life but the lives of hundreds of his trainees. From the dazzling way adrenaline controls critical body functions to the thrill of his Nobel Prize win, this engaging book will help you better understand how physician-scientists dedicate their careers to understanding human biology and enhancing human health."

—**P. Roy Vagelos, M.D., Retired Chairman and CEO, Merck & Co.; Chairman of the Board, Regeneron Pharmaceuticals**

"A blend of comedy, history, and tragedy, this book is much more than a delightfully amusing tale of a bright kid from the Bronx who ultimately wins a Nobel Prize. Bob Lefkowitz's message is of the utmost importance. U.S. taxpayer dollars funded a unique cadre of young physicians—'the Yellow Berets'—whose discoveries have led to revolutionary therapies for heart disease, cancer, diabetes, impotence, neurodegeneration, HIV, and coronavirus, all while training the next generation of medical scientists. Reading this book shows that investments in science will continue to save the world."

—**Peter Agre, M.D., Professor and Director, Johns Hopkins Malaria Research Institute, Bloomberg School of Public Health; Nobel Prize in Chemistry (2003)**

"A spell-binding memoir, packed with deep insights and charged with the thrill of discovery. This is a tale told from the pinnacle of human achievement, that also serves as a master-class in humility and overcoming tragedy—all interwoven with laugh-out-loud anecdotes. Lefkowitz is a brilliant and charming storyteller, with an indomitable passion for living, and wisdom for the ages."

—**Karl Deisseroth, M.D., Ph.D., Stanford University, Winner of the Kyoto Prize and the Heineken Prize; Author of** *Projections*

"Robert Lefkowitz's memoir is a rollicking, absorbing read. It turns out many funny things happened on his way to Stockholm. Beautifully written, this book demonstrates the importance of humor, humility, and humanity in the pursuit of scientific discovery."

—**Jerry Speyer, Chairman, Tishman-Speyer**

"An incredible story from one of the nation's finest scientists. Bob Lefkowitz is a true national treasure (and a real mensch), and this book is for anyone who wants to see how the extraordinary mind of a Nobel Laureate works."

—**David Rubenstein, Chairman Emeritus, Duke University Board of Trustees; Co-Founder, The Carlyle Group**

"A deeply personal perspective of events, people, thoughts, and actions that have created an era of major scientific breakthroughs. Full of insights and revelations about the milieu that underlies today's biomedical revolution, from a key participant. Written with a candor and style that make Bob Lefkowitz's life adventures as a physician-scientist a delight to read."

—**Stanley N. Cohen, M.D., Professor of Genetics and Medicine, Stanford University**

"Lefkowitz provides joyous remembrance of his amazing career as a physician-scientist. Interlaced with vignettes of personal sacrifice, growth, and friendship is the story of the seminal discoveries that culminated in science's highest award. A beautiful story of family, hard work, and steadfast optimism."

—**Christine Seidman, M.D., Professor, Harvard Medical School, Director, CV Genetics Center, Brigham and Women's Hospital**

"Bob Lefkowitz is a legend in his own time. In addition to his clinical background as an MD and acknowledged scientific mettle resulting in a Nobel Prize, he is a renowned raconteur. Bob also has an excellent sense of humor, and these twin skills have made him a highly sought-after public speaker. They are both on vivid display in this highly readable and entertaining autobiography, which begins with his childhood in the Bronx and embraces his long and distinguished career."

—**Michael Rosbash, Ph.D., Peter Gruber Professor of Neuroscience, Brandeis University, Investigator of the Howard Hughes Medical Institute; Nobel Prize in Physiology or Medicine (2017)**

"Lefkowitz is not only a gifted scientist, but also a gifted story-teller. From the Yankees to Duke basketball to the game show *Jeopardy!* through the upper echelons of science on his way to a Nobel Prize, he proves that science can be fun and rewarding for himself, the field, and his patients."

—**Brian Druker, M.D., Director, Knight Cancer Institute, Oregon Health & Science University**

A Funny Thing Happened on the Way to Stockholm

A Funny Thing Happened on the Way to Stockholm

The Adrenaline-Fueled Adventures
of an Accidental Scientist

Robert Lefkowitz, M.D.
with Randy Hall

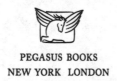

PEGASUS BOOKS
NEW YORK LONDON

A FUNNY THING HAPPENED ON THE WAY TO STOCKHOLM

Pegasus Books, Ltd.
148 West 37th Street, 13th Floor
New York, NY 10018

First Pegasus Books cloth edition February 2021

Interior design by Maria Fernandez

Library of Congress Cataloging-in-Publication Data is available.

ISBN: 978-1-64313-638-7

10 9 8 7 6 5 4 3 2

Printed in the United States of America
Distributed by Simon & Schuster
www.pegasusbooks.com

For all those who have taught and inspired me,
especially my parents, my wife Lynn, my children, and my students.

CONTENTS

	Preface	xiii
1	Matters of the Heart	1
2	Young Man in a Hurry	7
3	The Mysteries of Medicine	15
4	"Who's in the House Tonight?"	27
5	The Yellow Berets	38
6	Breaking the Rules at Mass General	52
7	"Duke? I Never Heard of It."	65
8	Travelin' Man	76
9	Learning to Say No	85
10	The Howard Hughes Medical Institute	90
11	Two Thousand Frogs a Week	98
12	"Mystery Physician Saves Man's Life"	110
13	The Quest for the Holy Grail	123
14	The Rosetta Stone	136
15	How to Fix a Broken Heart	148
16	Against the Odds	158
17	"Well, It's Not the Nobel Prize . . ."	167
18	*Jeopardy!*	177
19	The International Scientific Prize Circuit	186
20	The Death Project	197
21	Eat More Chocolate, Win More Nobel Prizes	208
22	Nobel Week	220
23	The New Normal	239
24	The Art of Mentoring	249
25	Roots	262
	Notes	269
	Acknowledgments	303
	Index	307

PREFACE

Anyone who knows me appreciates that everything reminds me of a story. As I have gotten older, there has been a rising chorus of trainees, colleagues, and friends who have urged me to write some of my stories down. Frankly, I never thought that I would. But then Randy Hall, who had done a postdoctoral fellowship in my lab during the '90s, and who is now a professor of pharmacology at Emory University, came to me with an interesting proposal. I had kept up with Randy over the years, as I do with many of my former trainees. Randy is a die-hard Duke basketball fan and was visiting Duke to attend a game with me during the 2018–2019 season. As usual, over a pregame dinner, I was regaling him with stories.

"Bob," he said, "I've got an idea that I would like you to consider. How about you start telling me your stories, I'll record them, write them up, and then you can edit the text?" Randy cited the best-selling book by the Nobel Prize–winning physicist Richard Feynman, as told to his friend Ralph Leighton (*"Surely You're Joking, Mr. Feynman!"*), as an example of this genre. And so the idea for this book was born. Over the next year we talked an average of one to two hours each week, with me telling my stories roughly chronologically, from my early days growing up in the Bronx in the '40s and '50s right up until the present.

While the broad outlines of my science receive some mention throughout, this is most certainly not a scientific autobiography in any conventional sense. If anything, descriptions of my research serve more as a scaffolding on which to hang stories of my adventures, with the more complex scientific material and references presented in chapter endnotes so as not to interrupt the flow of the main narrative. The telling of these tales has been a true collaboration between Randy and myself. Sometimes the voice is entirely mine, and sometimes it may be more of a hybrid between our two voices. However, all the stories represent my best recollection of events as they happened. Fully aware of the fallibility and malleability of human memory, I anticipate that some of those involved in the incidents recounted here may have slightly different recollections of certain events, and I alone bear responsibility for any errors. In situations where my interactions with patients are described, identifying details have been either changed or omitted to protect patient privacy.

Not to get too circuitous, but a major recurring theme of the stories told in this book is my love of listening to and telling stories. In fact, it wasn't until I began working on this book that I realized just how central stories and storytelling have been to my entire life and career. As a youngster, I read voraciously and even faked illnesses to stay home and read books. As a physician, I learned how to elicit a detailed history of a patient's illness and weave a story that would lead to the most likely diagnosis. As a scientist, I learned that data alone have little meaning until we impart it through narratives that are creatively constructed—based on the data—to yield some sort of conclusion or finding. As a mentor, I always take great interest in the stories of my trainees' lives, and often illustrate key points (both scientific and philosophical) by telling stories.

I am blessed to have lived a remarkably full, privileged, and fulfilling life. When I speak to students about my career, I sometimes use the title "A Tale of Two Callings," which refers to my sequential vocations, first the practice of medicine and then the pursuit of scientific research. I experienced each as something I was destined to do, and I have absolutely loved working at the intersection of these two unique worlds, as I hope will be apparent in these pages. Despite the fact that much of this narrative is lighthearted and humorous, there are also more serious undercurrents, including my decades-long battle with coronary artery disease, a bequest from both of my parents. I hope that many readers may learn something useful from the lessons and perspectives that I have gained as a "physician-patient." I cannot imagine a more rewarding career than being a physician-scientist and having the opportunity to help patients at the bedside while also making discoveries in the laboratory that lead to novel therapeutics. I hope that appreciation is evident in these pages.

ONE

Matters of the Heart

I was starting to get loopy from the drugs. My friend Dave stood over me, wielding a giant needle.

I lay on an operating table in the Duke hospital, undergoing a procedure to visualize the arteries that supply blood to the heart. Dave was a colleague of mine, so I knew I was in good hands. In fact, as a member of the Duke Cardiology faculty myself, I knew and trusted every single person in the room. At that moment, though, my faith in their expertise brought me little comfort.

For months, I had been feeling pressure in my chest after running or other exercise. As a cardiologist, I should have instantly recognized this feeling as angina. However, I employed an elaborate scheme of denial to convince myself otherwise. I was holding out hope that I was just a fifty-year-old guy experiencing muscle tightness or some other minor ailment.

As the symptoms persisted, I finally had a frank discussion with a colleague who convinced me to stop ignoring the obvious and get my heart checked. And so I found myself on the operating-room table, where Dave was now inserting a needle into an artery in my thigh, injecting a dye that would reveal what was going on. My heart was already being imaged on the screen in front of me, so despite my increasing sedation I could clearly see its contours.

Immediately, and with terrifying clarity, I saw segments of my coronary arteries lighting up in a way that revealed grave clogging.[1] The sedation was kicking in and I felt myself drifting off to sleep, but I managed to utter two last words before losing consciousness.

"Oh shit."

◆

My father had his first heart attack when he was fifty years old. I was twelve at the time. Nobody enjoys feeling like they're turning into their parents, but in this case the parallels between my father and me were obvious. I was on the same path that led to my dad dying young.

My father's heart condition colored my entire childhood. After that first heart attack in 1955, he spent three weeks in the hospital. When he finally returned home, his doctor told him to avoid all strenuous activity. This advice is ironic in retrospect because it's the exact opposite of how we advise cardiac patients today. Regular exercise is now proven to help prevent the reoccurrence of heart attacks. In those days, though, cardiac patients were told to avoid any activity that might raise heart rate, so that's what my father did.

When we would go on vacation, I would always carry the suitcases so that my father could take it easy. Whenever anything heavy needed to be lifted around the house, my mother asked me to do it, because Dad had a heart condition. My father no longer played sports with me after his heart attack. Our relationship was fundamentally altered, and I felt wistful about the many activities I could no longer pursue with the man I so worshipped.

My father's heart troubles also exacerbated my mother's anxiety. My mother was a nervous Nellie who worried about everything. My father came home every evening at 7:00 P.M. from his job in the Garment District of New York City, and if he wasn't home by 7:05 my mother would get visibly anxious. She imagined all sorts of horrible scenarios: he had keeled over on the subway because of his heart, or maybe he'd been hit by a train.

To help deal with her anxiety, my mother had been prescribed a medication called Miltown. It was a green liquid that was a forerunner of later anxiety drugs such as Valium. My mother referred to Miltown as her "green medicine," and she would swig it directly from the bottle like it was whiskey from a flask.

"Aren't you supposed to take a certain dose of that?" I once asked her as a kid. She fixed her gaze on me.

"I take what I need."

Whatever its anxiolytic effects, Miltown never dulled my mother's oversight of my daily activities. I was constantly in trouble with my mother, usually for good reason. In elementary and middle school, I would often play hooky, telling my mother I had a stomachache. Then I'd lie in bed all day reading books. During those long, lazy reading days, I would also cut coupons out of the *New York Times* book review section and order more books. I recall ordering Winston Churchill's six-volume *The Second World War* and Carl Sandburg's six-volume *Abraham Lincoln: The War Years*. I loved those books and read them cover to cover. Of course, ordering these book sets via the Literary Guild and Book of the Month clubs obligated my parents to buy large numbers of additional books. When my mother received notices in the mail about her financial obligations due to book sets ordered in her name, she suspected me immediately and started raking me over the coals like an FBI agent grilling a mobster. I tried to plead ignorance at first but ultimately wilted and confessed under my mother's withering cross-examination.

Even tougher than my mother's interrogation technique was her drill-sergeant-like attitude toward my piano lessons. I hated playing piano and would time my practices for when I knew my mother was going out for errands. We lived in the Bronx in a small rent-controlled apartment, right near the elevator. I would begin playing just before my mother left and then listen for the elevator bell. As soon as I heard that bell, meaning my mother had gotten on the elevator, I would get up from the piano and go hang out with my friends down the hall.

I worked this ruse for months, but then one day disaster struck. My mother went out the door, the elevator bell rang, and I got up from the piano. Just to make sure my mother was gone, I went over to the door and looked out the peephole. My mother's eye was staring right back at me! She had pressed the elevator button but then stayed by the door to spy on me. She came back inside screaming and stood resolutely behind me for the rest of the practice session.

In addition to playing piano for my mother, I also played regularly for less critical audiences comprised of my aunts, uncles, and cousins. I played terribly, of course, because I didn't practice enough. My mother would be openly disappointed in me, but nonetheless I loved these occasions when my extended family would get together. I was an only child, so I reveled in the chance to hang out with all of my cousins. Like many immigrant Jewish families who came to New York City during the migration from eastern Europe, my extended family regularly assembled for large gatherings of the entire clan. This "cousins club" in which my family participated was known as the AKD's, which stood for "Associated Kremsdorf Descendants" (Kremsdorf being the maiden name of my paternal grandmother). Every AKD gathering began with a business meeting, which was followed by a potluck supper and then a social hour in which the kids would perform for the adults. These get-togethers were extraordinarily well organized: we had a constitution drafted by my Uncle Charlie, who was a lawyer, and the business meetings were conducted strictly according to Robert's Rules of Order. The family was divided into committees, which gave progress reports regarding their activities. We even had elected officers. My father served as president for four years during my childhood, which made me very proud.

My father was my hero. He would do absolutely anything for me. One time, I was struggling in gym class at school. The class included a series of fitness challenges, such as climbing a rope all the way to the top in a certain amount of time, and you had to pass these challenges or else you would fail the class. I would strain on the rope to the point of exhaustion but never get very far off the ground. Fearful of failing the class, I confided in my father. He bought a long rope, set it up on a tree, and cheered me on as I practiced climbing. He taught me how to twist the rope around my leg to climb higher. By the end of the term, I was such a strong climber that I actually looked forward to being tested. My father's attention to my development had a delightful combined effect: as he helped me build skills, he also helped me build confidence in my ability to succeed.

It turned out that my father helped me to develop lots of skills for the future. In particular, my passion for math emerged through games I would play with my father. My father was an accountant, and on Saturdays I would accompany him to his office in the Garment District, where he would balance the weekly books. My dad would challenge me to races: we would both add up long lists of numbers, and I was allowed to use an adding machine while my father just used his brain. He beat me every single time. He was remarkably nimble with numbers and taught me tricks for how to do numerical calculations quickly. These Saturday morning games instilled in me a lifelong love of math and moreover represented precious time with my father. Our mornings spent together became all the more precious to me after my dad nearly died from his heart attack.

We were lucky to have an extraordinary family doctor, Joseph Feibush. If there was any man I admired as much as my father, it was the man who was committed to keeping my father alive. Dr. Feibush would make house calls and seemed to know everything about everything. I was fascinated by his set of tools, especially his stethoscope, which he allowed me to use to listen to my own heartbeat. After my dad's heart attack, I especially treasured Dr. Feibush's comforting presence, as I saw him helping to keep my father well. I dreamed of becoming a physician myself and gaining the power to keep people's loved ones alive.

I yearned to become a doctor as soon as possible. Just as my father had given me the skills to scamper up the gym rope at full tilt and to calculate numbers with freakish speed, he had also prepared me to move at lightning pace on my academic path. I had developed into a master test-taker, blazing through answers using mental tricks learned from my father. I aced a standardized exam after sixth grade and was allowed to skip a grade, so I was progressing through my schooling much faster than normal. Then, in early 1956, I took another test that completely changed my life.

TWO

Young Man in a Hurry

I was a math and science nerd, and I yearned to be amongst others of my ilk. In New York in the 1950s, the school of choice for aspiring doctors, scientists, and engineers was the Bronx High School of Science. Admission to this specialized public high school was determined by a test that was open to every junior high school student in New York City. If you scored in the top eight hundred or so in the city, you were granted admission. There was no interview, no essay, no consideration of grades—just a test.[1] My father peppered me with practice questions to help prepare for this exam and I ended up making the cut, enrolling jubilantly at Bronx Science in the autumn of 1956.

Bronx Science was all the way across town from my apartment, so I took an elevated subway train to school each morning. I loved riding the train, watching the city rush past, feeling like I was hurtling into my future. The return trip each afternoon was also great, as the train tracks ran right past Yankee Stadium. If the Yankees were playing, you could watch the game while the train ran along the raised track beyond the outfield bleachers. Sometimes the conductor would slow the train, such that the view of the stadium lasted for a minute or longer. During this glorious minute, my friends and I would press our faces up against the glass to watch our heroes in action. I was a devoted Yankees fan and especially worshipped the Yanks' fleet star Mickey Mantle. Before I dreamed of being a doctor, I had dreamed of being the next Mickey, but my utter lack of hitting, fielding, and running abilities had convinced me that being the next Dr. Feibush was a more realistic career goal.

There were a lot of nerds at Bronx Science, and I certainly held my own among them. I wore thick glasses and was as skinny as a slide rule. My nerd quotient was further enhanced by the fact that my two best friends, Steve Rudolph and Gene Frankel, were also unabashed nerds. Steve was a chemistry prodigy who took a perverse delight in correcting chemistry teachers whenever they said something wrong,[2] and Gene was a physics enthusiast who had an unnatural obsession with the history of science.

Steve, Gene, and I bonded over our lack of romantic success, which we attributed entirely to our lack of muscles. The 1950s were an era in which muscle men were worshipped, and thus we concocted a plan to speed the development of our manly physiques in order to impress the ladies. We each obtained a set of weights and met several evenings per week on a rotating basis to pump iron together. We also obsessively read bodybuilding magazines to learn the most up-to-date workouts and technical tips.

Our plan went well until one evening in my apartment when I performed a snatch with too much weight and lost control of the bar as I thrust it into the air. The bar flew backward over my head and smashed like a wrecking ball into my bedroom wall, sending chunks of drywall flying in all directions. My mother was livid and confiscated my weight set the next day, which meant that all future weightlifting sessions had to be held at Steve's and Gene's places.

The weightlifting must have paid dividends, because in the summer after my first year at Bronx Science I got my first girlfriend. This long-awaited and miraculous event occurred at a summer camp in Monroe, New York. At the same camp the previous summer, I'd had a crush on a sweet, shy brunette named Arna. She had a boyfriend at that time, but I learned that she was now no longer with him. I began to talk to her more and realized that we had a lot in common. We were both Jewish and came from kosher homes, for starters, and we liked a lot of the same movies. Moreover, her father had died of a heart problem several years earlier, when she was ten years old. I powerfully connected with her when she told me this story, given my own father's brush with death around the same time. Arna confided that I was the first person to whom she had ever opened up about her father's death. In turn, I shared with her my bottled-up feelings about how my family life had changed since my father's heart attack.

When summer camp was over, I returned to New York City to continue at Bronx Science. Arna lived in White Plains, about thirty miles north of the city, and we stayed in touch by mailing letters back and forth. Long-distance phone calls were expensive in those days, so talking on the phone was not an option. I also had no car. However, Steve had a car, so I set him up with Arna's friend Barbara. My strategy worked to perfection: Steve and Barbara hit it off, and in fact later got married, which was great because it meant on weekends I could catch rides with Steve to White Plains. Steve drove a souped-up Chevy with giant fins, and we spent many Saturday afternoons roaring up the Bronx River Parkway at full tilt for date nights with our girlfriends.

I was more than happy having a long-distance relationship at this time because I was so intensely focused on my studies during the school week. I was challenged by my ultra-competitive peers at Bronx Science and also challenged by the school's many outstanding teachers. One of my English teachers, Mrs. Gordon, was feared throughout the school and took an especially tough line with me. She seemed to despise everything I wrote. When we were gearing up to take Advanced Placement exams, she went around the room predicting how every kid would do. What kind of teacher does that? The exams were graded one to five, with five being the best and qualifying for advanced college credit. Anything less than a five meant that you might not qualify for credit, depending on the college. For most kids in the class, Mrs. Gordon predicted a score of five. When she came to me, though, she gave a sour look and predicted a three. Needless to say, I prepared rigorously for the exam.

A week later, the AP grades were in and Mrs. Gordon read them out loud in front of the class.

"Glass, five. Johnson, four. Lefkowitz . . . five," she said in an exasperated tone. "Honestly, I don't know how you did it, Lefkowitz."

To this day, I have no idea whether Mrs. Gordon actually disliked me or was instead a genius motivator who realized that she could push my buttons by doubting my abilities. Of course, both of those scenarios could be true.

In addition to focusing on my coursework, I also served as a math tutor and mentor to several younger students during my last two years at Bronx Science. One of these students was Stokely Carmichael, who would later go on to achieve prominence in the civil rights movement. Stokely was one of just a handful of African American students at Bronx Science, which couldn't have been easy for him. When Stokely and my other mentees began thriving under my tutelage and acing their math tests, I felt more charged up about their success than I did about my own grades. It was my first taste of mentoring and I loved it.

◆

I graduated from Bronx Science at the age of sixteen with a passionate desire for two things: becoming a doctor as fast as possible and staying close to Arna. Attending Columbia University accomplished both of these goals. Columbia had a strong premed program and was located in the city, which was important because Arna still had two years of high school left.

I discovered whole new realms of New York City when I moved to Manhattan to attend Columbia. I would go out with friends in Greenwich Village to see avant-garde art shows and musicians. I'd catch performances by edgy comedians like Mort Sahl and Lenny Bruce. Even the act of studying seemed more glamorous in Manhattan, as I would hit the books many nights at the New York Public Library main branch on Forty-Second Street and Fifth Avenue, a grand old library with vaulted ceilings and spectacular reading rooms.

The Columbia faculty at that time included some of the most iconic public intellectuals of the twentieth century, such as the literary critic Lionel Trilling, the cultural historian Jacques Barzun, and the sociologist Daniel Bell. They spearheaded the Contemporary Civilization curriculum that was required of all students in the first two years. In the class I had with Bell, I wrote a term paper entitled "Comparison of the Theories of Class Structure of Karl Marx and Max Weber." I was very proud of this title, which I thought sounded deep.

When the term papers were handed back a week later, everybody except me received a grade. My paper had no grade, and at the top Bell had written "SEE ME."

"Okay, here's the problem I've got," Bell said when I showed up to his office hours. "I've read your essay several times. It's either one of the most insightful essays I've ever read by an undergraduate, or it's complete bullshit. I don't know which it is, but I thought if we talked about it for half an hour, maybe I could get a better feel."

And so the battle was joined. I realized that I needed to defend my essay or he might fail me. For half an hour, I bobbed and weaved and argued my case with all the highbrow jargon I could muster. Finally, we got to the end of the allotted time and Bell peered at me over his glasses.

"You know, Lefkowitz, I've enjoyed our chat but still have no idea whether or not you're full of it. So how about we call it a draw and I give you a B?"

"I'll take it!" I exclaimed as I jumped up from my chair, exhilarated at having survived this battle.

In my second year at Columbia, I missed several days of classes to visit home after my father had another heart attack. He spent three weeks in the hospital again, and when he was released this time the doctors put even more restrictions on his physical activity. Unbeknownst to me, I was laying the groundwork for my own cardiovascular problems later in life thanks to my diet in this era. I ate a huge plate of eggs every morning for breakfast and then usually had an egg salad sub later in the day. Several nights each week, I ate at Tad's Steaks. You could get a full steak dinner there for $1.19, which was dirt cheap even by the standards of that era. The low price was presumably a reflection of the paucity of actual meat, with the overwhelming mass of the "steaks" at Tad's being comprised of gristle. These daily doses of steak and eggs were setting the stage for my own cardiac problems down the road, but like everybody else in the world in the 1960s I was completely oblivious to the risks of too much saturated fat and cholesterol. Little was known at that time about the connection between high cholesterol and atherosclerosis, so I had no reason at all to even think about my diet.

My father's second heart attack renewed my sense of urgency about becoming a doctor. I was a young man in a hurry. After my second year at Columbia, I realized that I wasn't far from graduating. I had come into college with a number of credits from Advanced Placement courses at Bronx Science, and on top of that I had taken large course loads each semester. I calculated that if I took a few summer courses, I could graduate from Columbia after my third year and start medical school early. This goal drove me all through the next year.

I was also in a hurry in my personal life. Things were going well with Arna, and I decided in the spring of my third and final year at Columbia that I wanted to propose to her even though I was just nineteen and she was seventeen. There was only one problem: I had no money to buy an engagement ring. Shortly before graduation, I received a letter from the bursar informing me that there had been a mistake in the processing of my tuition and I had overpaid. This letter was accompanied by a check for $250. I didn't understand how I could have overpaid the tuition, but I wasn't going to question it. I decided to use this unexpected windfall to buy an engagement ring for Arna.

I went diamond shopping, but the diamonds I could afford for $250 were tiny shards, barely visible to the naked eye. I ended up buying her a pearl ring instead. When I pulled the pearl ring out of my pocket a few days later and popped the question to Arna, she accepted with a big smile, and we were officially engaged. Two days before graduation, though, I received a panicky phone call from the bursar's office informing me that the $250 tuition rebate I'd received had actually been intended for a different student on campus named Robert Lefkowitz. Where else but New York City could you have two Robert Lefkowitzes in one class? As improbable as the situation seemed, I now had to pay the money back or I would not be allowed to graduate.

I didn't have the money. I knew that my parents' financial situation was very tight, so I couldn't ask them to bail me out after I just blew a wad of cash on a ring. However, time was short and I had nowhere else to turn, so I called my father to ask for his advice. He said that he would pay the money back to Columbia. I told him no, but he insisted, saying that I should consider it a graduation present and everything would be fine as long as my mother never found out.

I was now engaged to my high school sweetheart and ready to pursue my dream of becoming a doctor. Arna was planning on attending New York University, so my medical school applications were focused on staying in New York City. Columbia was the best medical school in the city at that time, so when Columbia accepted me, the matter was settled. In the fall of 1962, I began medical school at Columbia at the tender age of nineteen.

THREE

The Mysteries of Medicine

I had yearned to attend medical school since the age of eight, knowing it would be challenging but yet not fully prepared for what lay ahead. In gross anatomy class in my first year, for instance, I recall slicing open my cadaver and noticing something strange. In the upper portion of the right lung, there was a large mass that was white and cheesy. The location and nature of this mass suggested it might be a tubercular lesion, meaning my cadaver might have had tuberculosis at the time of his death. I was fully gowned, masked and gloved, but nonetheless still concerned about handling this apparent tubercular growth, which conceivably could contain active bacteria. I raised my hand to call for my instructor, a senior professor of anatomy. He strolled over with a cigarette dangling out of his mouth.

"Let me have a look at that," he said, reaching his bare hands into my cadaver's lung cavity. He pulled out a chunk of the cheesy mass and twiddled it between his fingers. "Yeah, I think you're right, this is probably TB. Go ahead and prepare a slide so that we can examine it in the pathology lab." With that, he took another puff on his cigarette and sauntered away.

Such grotesqueries were a common occurrence in my first year. Nonetheless, medical school was everything I'd dreamed it would be. I loved the lore, loved the exotic knowledge, loved helping patients. I loved my classmates,[1] including the erudite Harold Varmus, who had one of the keenest intellects I had ever encountered. Unlike my headlong rush to medical school, Harold had taken a more circuitous route, including obtaining a master's degree in English literature from Harvard. In contrast to Varmus's buttoned-down brilliance, our class clown, Robin Cook, became infamous on campus when he snuck pornographic slides into a pathology professor's carousel before class, resulting in scandalous images popping up on the screen during lecture. This prank prompted the professor to storm out of the lecture hall and complain to the dean, who demanded to know the identity of the perpetrator. We were a tight-knit bunch, though, so none of us gave Robin up, despite the common knowledge that he was responsible.

In addition to loving my classmates, I also loved my classes. I was especially enthralled by my biochemistry class with Erwin Chargaff, who everyone thought was going to win the Nobel Prize for his contributions to understanding the structure of DNA. When the Nobel Prize was announced that autumn for Watson, Crick, and Wilkins, but not Chargaff, there was campus-wide outrage over this perceived snub, as if the Nobel Committee had wronged Columbia itself.

I even loved my tiny one-room apartment in Bard Hall. The room's lone window looked out over a spectacular view of the Hudson River and George Washington Bridge. Just across the river was New Jersey, and at night I could see Palisades Park lit up, with the Ferris wheel turning and roller coaster racing. I'd ridden that Ferris wheel and roller coaster on dates with Arna, so I found the view from my room a source of joy and comfort even when I was up late studying for exams.

Yet my first two years of medical school were not exactly untroubled. For instance, during a pathology lab in my second year, I became convinced I had leukemia. I had prepared a smear of my own blood and began to panic when I counted far too many white blood cells. Leukemia was the obvious diagnosis, and immediately I began to reflect on how weak and fatigued I had in fact been feeling lately.

My mind was immediately filled with thoughts about Arna. We had gotten married a few months earlier, and she was now pregnant with our first child. What would happen to my wife and unborn child if I died from leukemia? Would I even get to meet my child? For years I had been worrying about developing heart disease like my father, but now suddenly it was clear I was going to die from leukemia well before heart disease could get me.

Terrified, I called over the instructor to confirm the diagnosis. Instead of offering consolation, though, he laughed in my face and told me I'd prepared the slide wrong. I was still in shock as the instructor patiently demonstrated the proper technique for preparing the slide, and soon I realized that my blood count was completely normal.

I had always been a bit of a hypochondriac, but now my medical studies were exacerbating this condition. Every weird disease we studied, I began feeling the symptoms. This worsening of my tendency to obsess over my own health was the only negative part of my medical school experience. I spent the first two years of medical school lurching from one false alarm to another.

Of course, some crises occurred that were not false alarms. I was doing a clinical rotation one day in the ER of the Columbia-Presbyterian Medical Center when the doors flew open and paramedics rushed in wheeling a blood-soaked patient.

"It's Malcolm X!" someone yelled.

The controversial leader of the Nation of Islam had been speaking across the street at the Audubon Ballroom when he was shot. As the paramedics sped past me, it was obvious that Malcolm was in bad shape. I leapt into action, prepping bags of saline and other items that might be needed in the ER suite. I then watched as the ER doctors worked on him in a frenzy of focused activity.

While craning my neck to get a view of what was going on, I began reflecting on the incredible unrest that America was undergoing at that moment in the country's history. A little more than a year earlier, I had been in my first-year physiology class when a student burst in and shrieked, *"President Kennedy has just been shot!"* Every person in the class immediately bolted out of their seats and headed to the nearest television set to watch the coverage. Now I was witnessing the attempted assassination of yet another major American political figure, except this time I was experiencing it in person and in real time. The scene was so dramatic, the tension in the air so palpable, I felt like I was watching a movie, except in this case I was *in* the movie.

After a short time, the turmoil quieted and the ER team emerged dejected. Malcolm had been all but dead on arrival, and there was nothing they could do. The ER went from chaotic to eerily quiet. Feelings of helplessness are common in medicine, but as the ER paused in that moment, our defeat was a heavy burden to bear.

◆

I learned a critically important lesson about medicine during my third year while doing a clinical rotation at Mount Sinai Hospital. My attending physician was a portly, affable pulmonologist named Mortimer Bader. During rounds at teaching hospitals, trainees typically gather the facts of a given case, including the patient's history, lab test results, and data from the physical, then present a narrative to the attending physician. Differential diagnoses are discussed and treatment plans are considered. In an early case that we handled on rounds with Dr. Bader, one of the other trainees presented a narrative about a patient with a lung problem, painting the picture of what seemed like a probable case of a life-threatening pulmonary fibrosis.

"Okay, good job," said Bader. "Now, Lefkowitz, I want you to use the same facts of the case, but tell me a different story."

I was dumbfounded. What other story could there be? The narrative presented by the other medical student seemed to fit all the facts. I hemmed and hawed, so Bader asked others in the group if they could tell a different story. Nobody was brave enough to try. Finally, Bader sighed and began to weave a story himself. Bader's gripping narrative was even more compelling than the first story, yet it painted a picture of a case of chronic asthma, a much less grave condition than pulmonary fibrosis. He had not changed any of the objective facts of the case; the only differences came from where he placed the emphasis and how he ordered the facts. When Bader was done, I suddenly felt confused about the case and realized that several more tests would be needed to truly figure out what was going on. Bader seized the opportunity to make a point about the importance of narrative in medicine.

"Many people think data tell a story, but nothing could be further from the truth. Data are just data. A *story* is something you impose on the data."

I was awestruck by this insight. I realized that I needed to open my mind and develop the ability to find multiple narratives in my patients' data, possibilities that could then be tested in order to arrive at the best diagnoses possible. Later in my career, when I became a serious researcher, Bader's insight about the importance of narrative would be even more valuable. Research often yields reams of data, which comprise the raw materials from which rational stories must be fashioned to explain how the world works. Of course, I had no interest at all in research during my medical school days. I was determined to become a practicing physician, and research seemed like a distraction from my single-minded goal.

I did have one brief exposure to research during medical school, and it did not leave a positive impression. After finishing the formal coursework in the first two years of the curriculum, I won a prize for having the best grades in my class. This prize, which was sponsored by the drug company Roche, consisted of a swanky new wristwatch and an all-expenses-paid trip to an exotic location: New Jersey. Specifically, I won a day at Roche's US headquarters in Nutley to see how drugs were developed. During this visit, I observed a team of Roche scientists who were searching for new cough medications. Their job was to screen every drug made in any program at Roche for the ability to suppress coughing, because cough suppressants were big moneymakers.

This research group's main experimental technique was to use a Rube Goldberg–type contraption to tickle cats' throats to induce coughing, then inject the cats with dozens of different drugs, one by one, to search for drugs that might reduce the feline hacking. I tried to hide my disgust from the researchers who were hosting me, but I was absolutely mortified by these studies. I felt sorry for both the cats and the poor bastards who had to spend all day tickling their throats. After this experience, I became even firmer in my conviction that I would never go into research.

I was equally sure that I would never become a surgeon. I greatly admired the surgeons I knew, but simply didn't possess the type of manual dexterity required for that line of work. In my fourth year of medical school, I did a sub-internship at a hospital in Cooperstown, New York. During this sub-internship, I enjoyed several visits to the Baseball Hall of Fame but found no joy at all in my required service assisting with surgeries in the hospital's operating room. During one procedure, the surgeon asked me to close up an incision with a few stitches, and I accidentally stitched my glove to the patient's abdomen. I had to get bailed out by one of the nurses, earning a scowl from the surgeon. Later,

I cut a deal in which I would no longer be involved with surgeries, which was in everyone's best interests. Instead, I would work extra shifts on the wards managing medical problems such as electrolyte imbalances and cardiac arrhythmias that arose in post-op patients, a duty that most of the surgeons despised but I loved.

The only thing I loved more than poring over patient data was chatting with the patients themselves. I loved taking patient histories—story after story for me to meld with data—and worked hard to cultivate my skills in this area. I was also fascinated by how dramatically my attitude and confidence could impact patient outcomes. In the final months of my training, I was doing a sub-internship at Goldwater Memorial Hospital, a chronic-disease center located on an island in the middle of the East River. This hospital was home to numerous patients who stayed there for months or years, with their care being supervised by generations of Columbia Medical students. During my time at Goldwater, I began treating an elderly woman who was suffering from chronic deforming rheumatoid arthritis. The only treatments available for this condition at the time—gold, corticosteroids, or high-dose aspirin—had all been tried with this patient but discontinued due to severe side effects. The woman was in an enormous amount of pain that could not be alleviated by morphine or other opiates because she'd also had bad reactions to these drugs. She begged me for something to ease her suffering.

"Well, as a matter of fact, we do have a new experimental drug that just came in, and it's supposed to be even more powerful than morphine," I intoned in a low voice, as if sharing a secret. "Do you want to try it?"

"Oh yes, I'm willing to try anything, doc" she replied. I prepared a syringe with a small amount of saline solution, but no drug.

"This drug needs to be given by needle, so you'll feel a small pinch. The drug should take effect in five or ten minutes," I said. I gave her a simple subcutaneous injection of saline and walked away to attend to other patients.

I was trying to harness the awesome power of the placebo effect. I had read the literature in this area and talked with several of my mentors about it, and I was fascinated by how a patient's belief in a treatment could strongly influence the eventual success or failure of that treatment. In my view, many Eastern medicine traditions were primarily predicated on the placebo effect: if a charismatic shaman gives a patient a nasty-smelling herbal preparation that has been used for centuries, there's a good chance that the patient will buy into the therapy and begin to feel better. I was hoping to take advantage of this effect to garner at least some measure of improvement for my patient with the severe rheumatoid arthritis.

When I came back around the ward to see her an hour later, the woman was effusive. She grabbed my arm and spoke in an ecstatic tone.

"Doctor! This new drug you gave me is amazing! I've got no pain at all! How much of this drug do you have? Can we get more?" I assured her that we had access to a large supply of the drug, then continued giving her once-daily saline injections for the next few weeks. She reported being completely free of pain and talked a blue streak about how she felt so proud to be the first patient in the hospital using this groundbreaking new drug. When my sub-internship ended, I made sure that the person who followed me knew all about this miraculous therapy that was so effective at treating the woman's pain.

As graduation neared, I received bad news: my father had suffered another heart attack. This news of my father's third coronary induced a flare-up of my own hypochondria, especially because my mother had also had a heart attack the previous year. I realized that I had bad genetics working against me on both sides of my family. I also now had medical training to make my concerns more concrete. I began noticing that my heart was prone to premature beats, resulting in a transient irregular heartbeat and fluttering sensation in my chest. I performed extensive experiments on myself where I would sit in different positions while tracking my heartbeat, hoping to find an optimal position for stabilizing the rhythm of my heart. However, weeks of self-experimentation resulted in no progress and no insights. I also had a full cardiac work-up, including an EKG, but the cardiologist said my heart looked normal except for the occasional premature beat. These optimistic words from the cardiologist did little to decrease my paranoia. I was convinced that heart disease was coming for me, just as it had come for both my parents.

The best remedy for my cardiac concerns was spending time with my growing family. Arna had given birth to our son David during my second year,[2] then became pregnant again soon after and gave birth to our second son, Larry (later to be known as Noah) during my last year of medical school. I was twenty-two years old, dirt broke, and the father of two. During that final year, I lived with my wife and two sons in a tiny one-bedroom apartment in the Bronx. This apartment was barely large enough for a single person to live comfortably, let alone a family of four. The tight squeeze was just fine, though—I loved my two little boys, so the cramped quarters and sleepless nights seemed like small prices to pay.

◆

As medical school wound down in the spring of 1966, my family's future was endangered by a looming threat: the Vietnam War. At that time, all graduates of American medical schools were required to enter the military to serve a year in Vietnam. There was no lottery system in this "doctor draft"—the military had an acute shortage of doctors, so *every* medical school graduate was mandated by law to serve. I believed in the importance of serving one's country but also dearly wanted to avoid being separated from my young family and sent halfway around the world for a year to support a war that I and most of my classmates believed was wrong. I felt a growing sense of trepidation and searched for some kind of alternate path that might allow me to serve honorably and also stay close to my family.

There were several ways for doctors to avoid serving in Vietnam. Medical school graduates were allowed to request a one- or two-year deferment to complete their internships and up to one year of residency training. After that, though, service in Vietnam was required unless some other arrangement was made. One attractive possibility was to gain a commission in the United States Public Health Service (USPHS), which was considered part of the US military and thus fulfilled one's draft obligation. USPHS physicians could work as prison doctors in the federal penitentiary system, help to track global pandemics at the Centers for Disease Control, or conduct research at the National Institutes of Health (NIH). Despite my previous lack of interest in research, I decided to pursue this last option.

I hoped to become an academic physician, maybe even a chair of Medicine at a top medical school someday, and was becoming aware that such positions required at least some research experience. Most of the prominent doctors who trained me at Columbia were alleged to have done research at some point in their pasts, and a handful were even supposedly still active. For example, one of my attending physicians, William Manger, was a subject of fascination amongst the medical students. Whenever he walked past, you'd hear people say in hushed tones, *"I hear he does research."* It clearly gave him a special cachet and cool factor.

Manger was also notable because he was the heir to a hotel fortune. He dressed sharply in three-piece suits, complete with a pocket watch dangling on a gold chain. Late in my last year of medical school, he invited several of us who were on rounds with him over to one of the Manger hotels downtown. After we enjoyed lunch in the luxurious dining room, Manger casually asked, *"Would you like to see my laboratory?"* We were curious, of course, and even more curious when he got into the elevator and pressed the button for the penthouse. When the elevator doors slid open, we strode into a spectacular suite that had been converted into a research lab. Hundreds of glass beakers were glinting in the abundant light, and the windows on all sides looked out over jaw-dropping views of New York City. I was in awe, and began to think that maybe research wasn't so bad after all.

Having decided that a bit of research might be a nice addition to my resume, I submitted my application to the NIH. I was accepted for an interview and drove to Bethesda, Maryland, for my interviews on July 1, 1966. Unfortunately, the first of July also happened to be the start date for my internship at Columbia-Presbyterian Medical Center. As if beginning my internship wasn't stressful enough, I had to miss my first day (and beg someone to cover for me) in order to conduct my interviews in Bethesda.

The interview process was a match-based system: applicants had to rank the group leaders with whom they wanted to work, and the group leaders in turn had to rank all the applicants. It was a highly competitive process, with hundreds of the best and brightest young doctors across the country applying for a limited number of slots.

My interviews at the NIH went poorly. For one thing, I had no research experience at all, which I began to realize was a major negative when interviewing for a research position. I had to explain over and over again to different NIH scientists why I hadn't bothered to take advantage of the various research opportunities that had existed at Columbia. My lack of research experience was compounded by my lack of enthusiasm, as I wasn't actually very excited about research but rather just trying to bluff my way through the process by pretending to be enthused.

The toughest interview of the day was my last, with a tall, hyperkinetic scientist named Jesse Roth. He asked why I wanted to come to the NIH. I said the words I thought he wanted to hear.

"My goal is to become a triple threat: I want to be a great physician, great researcher, and great administrator."

"That's bullshit," Roth replied. "You'll never be great at all three. You have to choose. Which would you choose if you could only be great at one?"

I was taken aback by his tone and stammered my way through an incoherent answer. When I left Roth's office and staggered back to my car, I was certain that I'd screwed up and wouldn't receive an offer for one of these coveted positions. I felt an impending sense of doom that I would soon be torn away from my family and sent on a tour of duty in the jungles of Vietnam.

FOUR

"Who's in the House Tonight?"

I was driving my car in the dead of night and could not keep my eyes open. Having worked a twenty-four-hour shift at the hospital for the third time that week, and with two young children at home, I was operating on less than twenty hours of sleep for the entire week combined. I was an intern now, a member of the house staff at the Columbia-Presbyterian Medical Center, and the schedule was killing me. Just the week before, during a dinner at home with Arna and the boys, I had fallen asleep at the table and faceplanted into a plate full of mashed potatoes and peas. Now, as I sped home through the darkness on the West Side Highway, it felt good to just let my eyes drift closed to rest them for a few seconds.

Suddenly, I was jarred to consciousness by a loud bump. My car had drifted across the right lane and hit the curb. I rapidly spun the steering wheel to correct course and get back on the road. As I tried to get my bearings, and also pick up the stethoscope that had fallen from the pocket of my white jacket, a siren began to wail and blue lights flooded my rearview. I pulled the car over.

"Doc, what's going on?" the cop asked as he approached my car. "You were weaving all over the road back there. Have you been drinking?"

"Absolutely not, officer. I just worked a long shift at the hospital and I'm trying to get home to my family. Can't you cut me a break?"

"Sorry, doc, the law's the law. Your license, please." I handed the cop my driver's license and his eyes widened. "Lefkowitz, huh? You any relation to Louis Lefkowitz?"

The attorney general of the state of New York at that time was Louis Lefkowitz. He was no relation to me, as far as I knew. However, my grandfather, a hat maker from Poland, was, amazingly, also named Louis Lefkowitz. I answered the policeman honestly.

"Louis Lefkowitz? Yeah, he's my grandfather."

"Oh geez," said the cop. "Well, I guess there's no point in me giving you this ticket. Your grandfather will just have it tossed. Okay, doc, I'm letting you go with a warning. Please drive home carefully." And I did . . . thanking the gods of coincidence all the way.

The bone-crushing fatigue I was feeling that night was a constant in my life, but I was loving my internship nonetheless. I was a real doctor now, and it was a thrill to walk into the hospital every day knowing I was in charge of a whole roster of patients. It was also scary, because I was now the one who was supposed to know what to do in all situations. Fortunately, I worked with a number of senior nurses who were accustomed to breaking in new interns. If I was treating an injured patient in the ER but forgot to order pain relief, for instance, one of the nurses would gently prod me to make up for my oversight.

"Doctor, you'd like to give this patient some morphine, correct? Would five milligrams be about the right dose?"

"Yes, yes, very good," I'd say, feeling both sheepish and thankful in equal measure. I made numerous little mistakes in my first few weeks as an intern, but fortunately the talented professionals around me were able to compensate for my lack of experience. Some of my fellow interns made clear to the nurses that they did not appreciate being corrected, but I was always grateful for the help. I viewed these senior nurses like mentors, and appreciated the way they tried to instruct me without showing me up. Later in my career, when I became a mentor, I tried to take a similarly positive approach with my trainees, as I never forgot how much such encouragement meant to me when I was a struggling intern.

The stress of my internship was compounded by the deep concern I felt about my future. I waited each day for news about whether I would get a position at the NIH and avoid serving in Vietnam. Concern over my impending service weighed on me, although the hundred-hour work-weeks and constant stress of my hospital work kept my mind occupied. My chief resident, Bill Lovejoy, pushed the house staff mercilessly. Bill was a former Yale football player who cut an imposing figure as he strode the hospital wards. Despite his gruff exterior, he was one of the finest physicians I ever encountered, and I learned a lot about doctoring from him. Bill was tough as nails and prided himself on never sleeping. If I was working a late-night shift and tried to sneak away when things were quiet to catch a half-hour nap in the on-call room, Bill would tease me in front of the nurses. Looking back on that era, it seems ridiculous that the entire Columbia house staff was so deprived of sleep and half-functional most of the time. These days, hospitals have changed their rules and placed restrictions on the number of hours that interns and residents can work in a given week. In the 1960s, though, shunning sleep was a key rite of passage by which young doctors demonstrated their toughness.

I required prodigious amounts of coffee to stay awake most days, and the flood of coffee plus the nonstop stress wreaked havoc on my gut. I developed persistent diarrhea, which is never good, but is especially bad when patients are counting on you to deliver timely medical care. During long shifts tending to one patient after another, I couldn't possibly take time to run to the bathroom every fifteen minutes. To combat my GI troubles, I began self-prescribing a syrup called paregoric, which was a tincture of opiates. I would walk around the wards swigging it straight from the bottle, just as I had seen my mother do with her "green medicine." The paregoric worked wonders in terms of stopping the diarrhea, but also had the unfortunate side effect of completely paralyzing my gut. Nothing at all was moving through my GI tract anymore, and I developed excruciating cramps with a high fever.

I had to be admitted to the hospital as a patient, and Bill Lovejoy insisted on overseeing my care. He wasn't exactly a sympathetic caregiver, and kept reminding me that because of my stupidity another member of the house staff had to be in the house (i.e., on call) rather than enjoying a scheduled night off. Bill also enjoyed pointing out that the standard protocol for these types of gut problems was to perform a sigmoidoscopy to make sure there wasn't a blockage. In those days, sigmoidoscopies were not performed with thin, flexible filaments like they are today, but rather with solid steel rods that were profoundly uncomfortable as they probed the sigmoid colon.

"Hey Lefkowitz," Bill kept saying with a smile. "If you're not better in forty-eight hours, you're gonna be riding the silver pony!" Needless to say, I recovered rapidly. It wasn't a placebo, but something close to it!

Shortly after this incident, I got a brief respite from Bill. By tradition, there was one week every year when the chief residents of Columbia and Harvard traded places, with the goal of having an exchange of ideas and best practices between these two great medical communities. This year in particular was exciting, with Bill Lovejoy bringing his unique brand of tough love to Harvard, and Columbia welcoming Sam Thier, who was legendary for both his brilliance and his pugnaciousness.[1] Thier was known to take sadistic pleasure in putting interns in their places by showing them how little they knew. When Thier arrived, I found out I was assigned to be the first intern to go on rounds with him the next morning, and I was absolutely terrified.

One of the first patients we saw was a patient of mine with a rare kidney problem. Thier's specialty was nephrology, so he took a keen interest in the case. He examined the patient's chart and sneered.

"You're probably not aware, Lefkowitz, but last week there was a big review in the *New England Journal of Medicine* about cases like this," he said when we stepped out of the room. "This review showed clearly that treatment Y is better than treatment X, so I want to know why the hell you're pursuing treatment X with this patient."

As fate would have it, I had in fact read the review article to which he was referring, and I knew he had his information wrong. Less than a day earlier, I just happened to be perusing this issue of the journal, which was laying around in our house staff library, and I'd noted this article about the rare kidney disease that one of my patients had. I was certainly no great connoisseur of the literature at that point in my career, so it was just a stroke of random luck that I'd stumbled across this review article. Nonetheless, having read the article mere hours earlier, I knew for a fact that Thier had misremembered the conclusions of the article, and I told him so.

"Well, I'm sure you're wrong, Lefkowitz," he said with unshakable Harvard confidence. "Do you happen to have this issue of the journal around so we can settle this matter?"

Naturally, I knew right where the journal issue was, because I had just read it the day before. I brought the journal to him and watched the smug smirk dissolve from his face as he read over the abstract and realized that the study had in fact recommended treatment X, the treatment I was giving my patient. After this incident, I became concerned that Thier might now make my life a living hell for the rest of the week because I had shown him up, but in fact just the opposite happened. We went on rounds together several more times that week, and each time he delighted in telling the tale to the other house staff members who accompanied us.

"I was on rounds my first day here with this kid Lefkowitz, and he absolutely nailed me!" he'd say, roaring with laughter. "I had some information backward about a kidney treatment, and he really put me in my place." This incident gave me a great confidence boost and also heightened my reputation amongst my peers, who all took pleasure in seeing the swaggering chief resident from Harvard forced to back down.

After a week, Thier departed back to Boston, Lovejoy returned, and I kept waiting to learn whether my next move would be to the NIH or Vietnam. Finally, a phone call came for me at the hospital and someone yelled down the hall that it was from the NIH. I raced to the phone and picked up the receiver. The call was from Jesse Roth himself, and he wanted to know if I would be interested in joining his research group. I accepted on the spot and raised my arms in triumph when I hung up the phone.

That evening, I celebrated the news with Arna. Several months earlier, we had welcomed our third child, a daughter named Cheryl, and moved to a two-bedroom apartment in Yonkers. Family life was sweet, other than the fact that I was falling over from exhaustion when I came home from work most nights. I wanted to spend more time playing with my kids, but my insane work schedule and constant sleep deprivation were having adverse effects on my parenting. There was one incident, though, when my medical training did have a positive impact on my family.

My oldest child, David, who was then four years old, was sick in bed one morning with a fever. I checked in on him, then gave Arna a kiss and headed out the door to go to my next shift at the hospital. I stepped into my car, but then paused. David just didn't look right. There was something about him, especially his breathing. I pulled the key out of the ignition and walked back into the house. Arna nearly dropped her coffee mug when she saw me.

"Aren't you on duty in half an hour?" she asked.

"I'll get someone to cover," I said, picking up the phone and dialing the hospital. "I just want to sit with David for a while. He doesn't look right to me."

I sat on the edge of David's bed and took his temperature several times over the next hour. His fever was rising. Worse, his breathing was becoming more labored. I wasn't exactly sure what the problem was, but my medical intuition told me that something was wrong. I scooped David up in my arms and headed to my car. Arna's mother had just come over, so I asked her to stay home with our other two children. Arna placed a quick call to David's pediatrician to let them know we were coming and we jumped in the car.

It was a twenty-minute drive, and during the journey David's condition began to rapidly deteriorate. With Arna swaddling him in a blanket in the passenger seat, David's breathing was becoming increasingly difficult and he was getting blue in the face with cyanosis. I suspected he might have epiglottitis, an inflammation of the lid that covers the windpipe. Such infections are rare but potentially deadly because the inflamed epiglottis can totally block the trachea and prevent breathing if not treated immediately. David's condition was worsening by the minute and I could hear him gasping for air. Panicked, I stepped on the accelerator and began hurtling at top speed through the streets of New York City, weaving in and out of traffic and running red lights.

We arrived at Albert Einstein Medical Center, jumped out of the car in front of the main entrance, and raced inside. A nurse tried to stop us, yelling that the doctor was with a patient, but I ran past her and busted into the examining room with David in my arms. The pediatrician immediately saw that David's face was blue, and looked down David's throat for a few seconds to confirm that it was indeed epiglottitis. He paged an emergency procedure, and at once there was a flurry of activity with nurses and staff members sprinting at full speed as David was wheeled to an operating room down the hall. I ran to the operating room and was met there by the pediatric anesthesiologist, who had just arrived by rushing up the stairs and was out of breath as he spoke.

"I'm gonna take one shot at sliding a tube through his nose and down his throat, but it'll have to be a perfect shot because the opening left in his throat is so small," the anesthesiologist said. "If that doesn't work, we'll have to trake him." By "trake," he meant perform a tracheotomy, a dramatic surgery that would involve slicing open David's throat to insert a tube that would allow him to breath on a ventilator.

I was asked to step out of the room, which is a helpless feeling for a doctor whose son is in a life-or-death situation. Fortunately, the anesthesiologist was a wizard with the tube and managed to get it down the throat on the first try without the need to cut open David's neck. David then spent the next several days in intensive care while taking antibiotics to treat the infection.

While I sat vigil with David in the ICU the next day, I reflected on what had made me stay home the previous morning. David had basically just been a kid with a fever, and kids are always running fevers. However, if I had left and gone to work that morning like normal, David probably would have died. Every good physician has to develop a sixth sense about when things aren't right, and somehow that morning my sixth sense had told me to stay with David.

After taking a few days off to spend with David while he recovered, I returned to the wards for my final clinical rotation. In a few weeks, I would be driving my family to Maryland so that I could begin my fellowship at the NIH. The last rotation of my junior residency would be in Harkness Pavilion, a section of the Columbia Medical Center with private rooms where many of the wealthier patients were treated.

One of the most famous actresses in the world at that time was admitted to Harkness in the early days of my rotation. This actress had suffered several fainting spells, including one onstage during a performance on Broadway. The tabloids all ran front-page stories about her, saying that she was in the hospital being treated for "exhaustion." While the gossip columnists chattered about the impact of this episode on her career, I sat at her bedside and tried to figure out what was wrong with her.

We ran blood tests and diagnosed her with an extreme case of hypokalemic alkalosis. This meant that her blood was too low in potassium (hypokalemic) and too high in pH (alkalosis). Basically, her blood electrolytes were off-kilter. But the question was: why? There are a number of potential causes of hypokalemic alkalosis, and I took a detailed history from her in order to start crossing potential causes off the list. Hypokalemic alkalosis can be caused by certain drugs, but she insisted that she was not taking any of the drugs I mentioned. Another potential cause is too much licorice. I asked her several times if she had an affinity for licorice, or perhaps licorice-flavored cocktails, but she told me that in fact she hated licorice and hadn't eaten it in years.

For several days, I was mystified, as was the attending physician on the case, Stuart Cosgriff. He was one of the most distinguished physicians on the Columbia faculty at that time, a real doctor's doctor. Cosgriff advised me that we needed more information from the patient to help crack the case, and I told him that I would do my best.

I spent more time talking to the actress, trying to get her to open up. She had a young son, so we talked about our kids. We also talked about our mutual admiration for Robert Kennedy, the presidential candidate who had been tragically assassinated several days earlier. We talked about her hopes and dreams and her various upcoming projects. She told me about the intense pressure she felt every day as a public figure, and how the tabloids were always commenting on her weight. Then, she confessed that sometimes after meals she felt guilty about eating and made herself throw up. She also sometimes abused enemas as a weight-loss tactic. As it turns out, excessive vomiting and frequent enemas are known causes of hypokalemic alkalosis, so this revelation seemed to explain her condition. However, it wasn't until she began to trust me that she was willing to admit to these behaviors.

I was moved by her story, especially because she seemed like one of the nicest people on the planet. At the same time, I was completely shocked. I had never heard of someone intentionally throwing up after meals. This eating disorder would later be named bulimia,[2] but nobody in that era had heard of it, and we certainly weren't taught about it in medical school. Flying by the seat of my pants, I counseled the actress that she absolutely needed to stop throwing up after she ate and also to stop abusing enemas. If left unchecked, hypokalemic alkalosis can lead to heart problems, kidney problems, and eventually death. I told the actress that if she wanted to see her son grow up, she needed to take care of her own health, and that this behavior was a serious threat to her life. She received the message well, vowing to stop at once and thanking me profusely for listening to her and lending a sympathetic ear.[3]

When I presented the wrap-up of the case to Cosgriff, he was impressed. He noted that the rapport I had developed with the patient, especially my careful listening to her life story, was the key to solving the mystery. We then discussed other patients he was overseeing in Harkness, and he expressed concern about two patients in particular who were not doing well and would require constant monitoring. As he packed up his briefcase and prepared to leave for the evening, he turned to me.

"Who's in the house tonight?"

"Me," I replied. "I'm on duty all night and all day tomorrow."

"That's wonderful news," Cosgriff said. "I'll sleep well knowing that you're in the house."

These words from Cosgriff represented one of the peaks of my professional life to that point. The fact that this legendary physician trusted me with his patients was the highest accolade I could imagine. I felt like

I had really made it. Not only was I a doctor, but I was a *good* doctor. I had found my calling. Or so I thought.

Little did I know it at that time, but I was on the verge of developing an obsession that would divert me from the full-time practice of medicine and completely change the course of my life.

FIVE

The Yellow Berets

I stripped off my doctor's whites and threw them in the hamper. As I dressed in my civvies, I was overwhelmed with bittersweet emotions. It was the last day of my junior residency at Columbia, and I was leaving medicine behind for a two-year research stint at the NIH. I strode out of the main door of Harkness Pavilion onto Fort Washington Avenue, where Arna and our three children were waiting for me in a Dodge Dart that was overloaded with luggage. I climbed into the car, and we began the drive to Maryland.

I was twenty-five years old and had never lived anywhere except within a ten-mile radius of New York City. Have you ever left behind everything you've known? Have you ever set off on a journey feeling utterly uncertain about your future? That was how I felt driving out of the city that day.

By evening, we arrived in Rockville and I began to feel better. We moved into a townhouse with multiple bedrooms and a grassy backyard.

The space felt positively luxurious compared to our cramped quarters in New York. We also felt rich: as an intern I had made $4,000 per year, but as an NIH fellow I would be making $12,000 even though my schedule would be much more relaxed. I was sad to be leaving the day-to-day practice of medicine but already enjoying the perks of my new lifestyle, with the major perk, of course, being that I got to be with my wife and kids rather than 9,000 miles away in Vietnam.

The Public Health Service—commissioned officers of that era who served at the NIH were known as the Yellow Berets.[1] The sobriquet was a play on the Green Berets, with the color change meant to suggest we were too scared to fight. Avoiding service in Vietnam was not an act of cowardice, though. For most, it was an act of conscience. The war was immensely unpopular, and massive antiwar demonstrations in downtown Washington, D.C., were a common occurrence during my two years of service. Arna and I took our kids to several of these demonstrations, which we recognized as history in the making.

Young doctors across the country were desperate to avoid being shipped off to war, so the NIH had received thousands of applications that year for fewer than two hundred slots. The intense competition meant that those selected were the cream of the crop, and I felt honored to be part of this august group. One of the other Yellow Berets starting at the same time was my friend and medical school classmate Harold Varmus, and it was comforting to see at least one familiar face during my first week at the NIH.

As commissioned officers in the Public Health Service, we were given the rank of lieutenant commanders. A major perk of being active duty officers was that we could fly standby anywhere in the country for free, so long as we were wearing our uniform. However, the uniforms were expensive, so five of us chipped in together and bought a uniform to share. If one of us were traveling in a given week, that person would use the uniform to fly for free. The only downside to this plan was that the guys in our group were all radically different heights, which meant that the uniform pants were too long on some guys but preposterously short on me. Whenever I flew in my uniform, my pants looked like I'd pulled them up to ford a river.

The Yellow Berets were all medical doctors doing research fellowships, but we also performed clinical duties. We worked at the NIH Clinical Center, a building that was half research space and half hospital. As part of a rotation, every fifth night we would sleep in the hospital to attend to any medical emergencies that might arise. Most of the patients we saw in the Clinical Endocrinology Branch where I worked had been flown in from around the country with exotic endocrine disorders. My mentor, Jesse Roth, had developed the first radioimmunoassay for measuring growth hormone when he was a trainee in the lab of future Nobel Laureate Rosalyn Yalow and her research partner Solomon Berson. For this reason, many of the patients we saw had acromegaly, a disorder caused by excessive growth hormone levels, and Jesse was carrying out detailed studies of such patients as part of our inpatient service.[2] These patients were flown in from all around the country and had characteristic enlargements of certain features, such as their jawbones and hands. In addition to seeing patients, we also dealt with issues like the arrival of tissue samples that needed to be stored for analysis the next day. One night early in my fellowship, I received an unusual phone call while I was on duty.

"Are you the officer of the day?" asked the hospital operator.

"Yes," I said. She continued in an urgent tone.

"Code yellow!"

"I . . . I'm sorry, I don't know what that means," I replied. Most hospitals of that era had color codes, which varied by hospital. Code blue was usually a medical emergency, whereas code red typically meant a fire. I was not familiar, though, with code yellow.

"Haven't you read your staff manual?" she asked.

"Uh . . . no, I guess I haven't. I'm new here. Can't you just tell me what code yellow means?"

"I'm not supposed to say it over the phone," she said, sounding exasperated. "But . . . okay. Code yellow means animals loose in the building. The call came from the ninth floor."

Animals loose in the building? I had visions of rhinoceroses stampeding down the ninth-floor hallway. I hung up the phone and raced to the ninth floor, which was mostly dark and deserted. There was a light shining from a single room in the east wing. I tiptoed toward the room in a ninja-like crouch, ready for whatever I might encounter.

When I reached the open door and peered around the corner, I saw a lab technician on his hands and knees.

"Did you call about animals loose in the building?" I asked. He was startled and spun around quickly.

"Yes. I've been working with mice and two of them escaped."

I breathed a huge sigh of relief that we were dealing with mice and not something larger that I might have to tackle. I joined the technician in his mouse hunt for the next half hour. We never found the mice, but I did file a report the next day stating that I had responded to a code yellow and was successful in keeping the building safe.

Other than my occasional duties as the officer of the day, I was mainly focused on research. My early days in lab were a complete disaster. One time, I was pushing a glass pipet through a rubber stopper when the pipet broke and deeply gouged my forefinger. This accident occurred in the evening, after most hospital staff had gone home, so there were no other physicians available to suture the wound. I sprinted to the emergency room of the Clinical Center, blood trickling down my hand, and found a nurse who assisted me as I sutured my own finger. Due to the fact that I was in severe pain, not to mention one-handed and out of practice, I did a lousy job. The aftereffects of this botched surgery would plague me for years to come. The incision appeared to heal, but then mysteriously flared up again every few months. Eventually, it broke down and began extruding tiny pieces of glass, with an X-ray revealing numerous additional shards of glass still embedded. Finally, an experienced surgeon performed an additional surgery to clean things out, allowing the finger to fully heal.

I survived my early struggles with help from my mentor, Jesse Roth. He was a nonstop dynamo of positive energy who kept everyone in the lab pumped up. During one of my first days in the lab, my labmate Gary Robertson opened an envelope containing reviews of a manuscript that he and Jesse had submitted for publication. The reviews pointed out numerous flaws in the submitted work, with one negative comment after another, and Gary put his head down on his desk in despair. At that moment, Jesse bounded into the office and snatched the letter from Gary's desk.

"What's the matter with Gary?" asked Jesse.

"He just got the reviews back on his paper and they're terrible," I said. Jesse began speed-reading the letter, and a smile spread over his face. He put the letter down and began pumping Gary's hand.

"Mazel tov! This is wonderful news!"

"What are you talking about?" asked Gary. "They hated it."

"Hated it?" Jesse said with a laugh. "These are rave reviews! If we just do a few more experiments, this paper will be accepted no problem." Gary and I thought Jesse was crazy. However, it turned out that after Gary did another few weeks of experiments to address the reviewers' comments, the revised paper was accepted for publication, just like Jesse said it would be. This was my first lesson in how to read reviews and also how to address reviewers' critiques to get papers published.

Jesse thought everything was great. Whenever I showed him a piece of data, no matter how insignificant, he would bounce off the walls with excitement. I usually had to discuss my findings with him while speed-walking down the hallway because he was in constant motion.

"Let's walk and talk!" he'd exclaim as he hurried off to his next meeting, his mouth running a mile a minute with excitement over how I was on the verge of a major breakthrough. I'd walk away feeling high as a kite. Then I'd show the same data to my co-mentor down the hall, Ira Pastan, and he would shake his head.

"Jesse was excited about this? It looks like some sort of artifact. Did you do a negative control? Did you do a positive control? Did you do ANY control?" Ira was a serious soul who was more interested in scientific rigor than in fanning the flames of his trainees' excitement. Showing data to Ira was often a humbling experience, but he gave me meticulous training in the art of designing and interpreting experiments.

The project that Jesse and Ira had given me was to identify the receptor for a hormone known as ACTH, which is a key regulator of the stress response.[3] For this project, the first thing I had to do was label ACTH with a radioactive tag, then separate the labeled hormone from the unlabeled. In theory, this sounds easy, but in practice, it was a titanic struggle. I did battle on a daily basis with an old fraction collector that I would fill with test tubes to capture my various fractions of ACTH as they came off a column overnight in the cold room. The fraction collector would work perfectly whenever I was watching, but then malfunction as soon as I walked away, causing my precious samples to spill all over the floor. I grew paranoid that the fraction collector was out to get me.

One night, I stayed late in the lab to keep watch over the fraction collector. I sat vigil in the cold room, shivering despite my overcoat. After three hours, I pretended to leave, went out to my car, turned around, and came back to the lab hoping to catch the fraction collector in the act of ruining my experiment. No luck—it was running just fine. Satisfied that I had solved the problem, I went home and tried to get a few hours of sleep. The next morning, I came in to find my samples all over the cold-room floor again. Ultimately, I convinced Jesse to buy a new fraction collector, but by then I had wasted months on these efforts with no progress at all.

During Thanksgiving break, Arna and I drove with our kids back to New York City to visit family. I was silent on the drive, feeling depressed by my constant failure in the lab. I had never really failed in a sustained way at anything in my life, except for rope climbing in junior high, and even that I had ultimately mastered with assistance from my father. We arrived in New York in time for Thanksgiving dinner with my parents, and after the meal I sat down with my dad to confess to him how despondent I was feeling. He listened intently and then offered some sage advice.

"Look, Bobby, you've always wanted to be a practicing physician, right? This research thing is just a way of staying out of Vietnam. What the hell do you care if the research succeeds or not? Just keep your head down, do your time, and in eighteen months you'll be heading off to complete your residency and pursue the career you've always dreamed of. Everything's gonna be okay."

I felt lighter than air after chatting with my dad. He had a way of always making things better, and in this case I really needed to hear his words. When Arna and I drove back to Maryland a couple of days later, I was in a better frame of mind and feeling buoyant about my future.

Two weeks later, I was seeing a patient during my weekly half-day clinic when a nurse yelled that there was a phone call for me. I picked up the receiver and was surprised to hear the voice of my family's physician, Dr. Feibush.

"Bob, your father has had another heart attack. I'm at your parents' home and we're waiting for an ambulance. Your mother asked me to call you, but I don't want you to worry. Your father seems stable and you should be able to talk to him later today."

I went back to my clinic, but an hour later my mother called the same phone and was hysterical. My father had died in the ambulance. There had been a delay in the ambulance arriving, my father's heart had suddenly stopped and he never even made it to the hospital. I dropped the receiver and walked out of the clinic.

I needed to get home, get my family together, and drive to New York as soon as possible. In the Jewish faith, funerals must take place within twenty-four hours of death. However, I wasn't even sure how to get home to Arna because I was part of a carpool and hadn't driven that day, so I had no car. I went back to the office I shared with several other Yellow Berets and bumped into Harold Varmus, who jumped up from his desk when he heard the news and immediately volunteered to take me home. On the drive, Harold and I had an intense discussion about our parents, our families, and our futures. Harold was usually so serious and unemotional, but during that car ride he comforted me in a way that allowed me to focus on gathering my family and heading for New York.

After my father's funeral, I returned to work in Maryland but found myself falling into a state of depression. My research was a fiasco. I was homesick for New York. And now this central pillar of my life, my father, was suddenly gone. I mourned for him and in a sense also mourned for myself, feeling more certain than ever that my father's untimely death presaged my own early demise.

◆

I was desperate for something that might improve my odds of defusing the time bomb in my chest. Before my father's death, I had read a popular book about a new method for improving cardiac health. In the aftermath of his death, as my mind continually cycled back to my own cardiac situation, I picked up the book again and decided to follow its advice. The book was *Aerobics* by Dr. Kenneth Cooper. In the book, Dr. Cooper presented extensive data supporting a radical idea: aerobic exercise like walking or jogging could improve cardiac performance and protect the heart from disease. This notion seemed both outrageous and counterintuitive to me, as my father had been told by his doctors for years that he needed to *decrease* physical activity in order to protect his heart. Nonetheless, the data presented by Dr. Cooper were compelling, so I was moved to make a lifestyle change and start exercising.

Knowing little about athletic footwear, I bought some Hush Puppies to use for light jogging. I had actually tried jogging a few times in New York City, but the mean streets of New York in that era were not exactly conducive to people trotting around for leisure. In contrast, the tree-lined streets of Rockville were perfect for morning jogs, so after my father's death I vowed to begin a daily habit. At first, I couldn't even jog a half mile without stopping, but soon I was trundling along each morning in my Hush Puppies for several miles without a problem.

In addition to improving my health, these morning runs also served as important moments for me to meditate and work though the grief I was feeling over my father. I also grieved in the evenings, after the kids went to bed, and would often sit alone listening to sad music. This went on for months. To this day, whenever I hear a song by Judy Collins, it brings me right back to this era, and tears start welling in my eyes.

The other way I dealt with grief was by working hard in the lab. I continued having technical troubles, but then suddenly, a year into my fellowship, a miracle happened: my experiments started working. The essential insight that led to my success was that I needed to ask others for help instead of just struggling by myself. I had been pursuing a daunting task, trying to separate labeled ACTH from unlabeled ACTH based on the tiny size difference conferred by the label. However, neither of my advisers were chemists, and I had never done any research at all, so I was just flailing. Finally, I sought out several expert chemists on the NIH campus to ask their counsel. With advice from these sages, I tried different types of columns and also ran my columns in different ways until I finally got traction in achieving chemical separation of the labeled ACTH from the unlabeled.

Once I finally had some pure labeled ACTH, everything else moved with breathtaking speed. In short order, I showed that the labeled ACTH was biologically active, and then rapidly developed one of the very first assays for studying the binding of a hormone to its receptor. Later in my career, I realized that this is often how research works: you experience nothing but failure for weeks or months, and then suddenly you overcome a technical hurdle, like in this case finding the right chromatographic system to separate the two forms of ACTH, and suddenly everything starts moving like wildfire. These were heady months, as I felt intoxicated by the knowledge that I was exploring new realms of research where none had previously trodden.

Following this unexpected deluge of data, Jesse told me that it was now time to write some papers describing our findings. I had never written a paper before, so I didn't know what to expect. Gerald Levey had been a Yellow Beret in Jesse's lab for the two years before me and was now running his own laboratory in the Heart Institute. When I told him that I was ready to work on some papers with Jesse, he laughed.

"Good luck writing with Jesse."

"What do you mean?" I asked.

"Well, Jesse thinks he's the greatest writer in the world," Gerry continued. "But this is not a universally shared opinion. When we got back the reviews of the first paper I wrote with him, which took us more than twenty drafts, one of the comments was, '*This is without a doubt the worst-written scientific paper I have ever read.*'"

Jesse invited me to his apartment to write. We sat at his kitchen table, facing each other. He began dictating some opening sentences, and I was writing the words down with a pencil. After every single sentence, we stopped to argue. Having been forewarned by Gerry about Jesse's overconfidence in his writing skills, I wasn't going to just jot down Jesse's disjointed sentences verbatim. For countless hours, we battled word by word, paragraph by paragraph. Finally, we had a rough draft, which I took home to type up and share with our coauthors to get their input.

Jesse wanted to publish this first paper, reporting the radiolabeling of ACTH and binding to its receptor, in the prestigious *Proceedings of the National Academy of Sciences* (*PNAS*). I knew nothing about scientific publishing, so this choice of journal meant nothing to me. Moreover, I had no idea what the process was. I soon learned that the only way to publish in *PNAS* in that era was to have your paper communicated by a member of the National Academy. Jesse showed the paper to Ed Rall, the scientific director of our Institute, who read it and offered a few suggestions. He then showed the paper to James Shannon, a former director of the NIH and a National Academy member. Shannon accepted Rall's word that it was good work and communicated it to *PNAS*. Thus, the paper was published without ever having to go through a formal review process.

Our next paper did get reviewed and ultimately published in *Science*. This paper described the development of the "radioreceptor assay" for a peptide hormone, the first such assay that utilized the receptor for the hormone rather than an antibody, as in radioimmunoassay. This assay allowed us to accurately measure levels of ACTH in bodily fluids. We also wrote another paper about the binding assay using labeled ACTH, and this paper was accepted for publication by *Nature*. I had gone from being a complete failure in my research to having three papers published in the world's most prestigious scientific journals in the span of just a few months.[4] I also got invited to give several talks about my research. My first scientific talk ever was a presentation on the NIH campus invited by future Nobel Laureate Marty Rodbell, whose laboratory was just around the corner from ours.

It turns out that this presentation, the first of my life, changed the course of history. I talked to Rodbell's lab about my efforts to study the binding of 125I-ACTH to its putative receptor. Rodbell and his team, including research associate Lutz Birnbaumer, were much more interested in functional experiments assessing the ability of hormones like glucagon to regulate cyclic AMP levels. They harshly criticized my data, saying that their functional experiments were far superior to my binding assay approach because there was no way for me to know if the ACTH binding I was measuring actually represented binding to a functional receptor. I left their lab with my tail between my legs, feeling like maybe they were right and I was wasting my time.

A week later, I saw Lutz's name on the sign-up sheet to get 125I at our radiation core facility. The main use of this radioactive iodine was to perform hormone binding assays, so I grabbed Lutz the next time I saw him in the hallway.

"Hey Lutz, I saw you signed up for some 125I. What's up with that? I thought you guys didn't believe in binding assays."

Lutz shrugged his shoulders.

"Yeah, well, after your hearing your talk, Marty thought maybe we should see if we can measure glucagon binding to its receptor. If it works, it might complement our functional experiments."

A few months later, history was made. Lutz and Marty were indeed able to measure the binding of 125I-glucagon to cell membranes expressing the putative glucagon receptor. They furthermore observed that this binding decreased when they added the standard buffer used for functional assays, which included adenosine triphosphate (ATP). This led them to examine other nucleotide triphosphates, including guanosine triphosphate (GTP), which they found was *10,000 times* more potent than ATP in disrupting the 125I-glucagon binding.

This finding led them to speculate that there must be a GTP-sensitive factor linking activation of the hormone receptor to its downstream regulation of cyclic AMP levels. Years later, Al Gilman (another Yellow Beret) would purify these GTP-sensitive factors, which became known as "G proteins." Rodbell and Gilman shared the Nobel Prize for these studies in 1994. However, the road leading to the discovery of G proteins began when I shared my binding assay expertise with Rodbell's lab; the key data that led them to hypothesize about the existence of G proteins in the first place all came from binding assays. At the time, I had been under the impression that Lutz and Marty thought my binding assay approach was worthless, but it turned out that my findings inspired them to pursue a line of research that led straight to a Nobel Prize.

◆

With just weeks to go in my tour of duty at the NIH, Jesse implored me to stay.

"You can't leave now, Bob! You've got a tiger by the tail!" Jesse told me over and over again.

Nonetheless, despite Jesse's pleas and also despite my growing excitement about research, I felt it was time for me to go back to clinical medicine. In the last conversation I'd had with my father before his death, we had made a plan: I was going to finish my period of conscripted active duty at NIH and then go back to being a full-time physician. After my father's death, this plan felt like an immutable pact.

Given my family history of heart disease, I decided to focus on cardiology. In the spring and summer of 1969, I went for several interviews to determine my next steps. I interviewed at my alma mater, Columbia, about doing a cardiology fellowship, but they had filled all their cardiology slots for the next two years and said I would have to wait an extra year. I also interviewed at Massachusetts General Hospital, one of the main Harvard teaching hospitals and considered by many to be the top hospital in the country.

During my visit to Mass General, I had a fateful interview with Charlie Sanders, the head of the cardiac catheterization lab. I confided to him that I had always wanted to be a cardiologist. I told him my plan was to get away from basic research and focus on more clinically oriented studies of blood flow dynamics in humans, just as he did. He fixed me squarely with his gaze and spoke slowly in his Texas drawl.

"Lefkowitz, guys like me are a dime a dozen, but cardiologists like you who can do biochemical and molecular work are as rare as hen's teeth. You want my advice? Stick with your biochemistry and learn how to apply it to the cardiovascular system."

I hated to hear these words at the time because I had already decided to give up basic research. However, Sanders's statement would prove to be prescient. Following my interview, Mass General offered me a senior residency slot in medicine to be followed by a two-year cardiology fellowship, which I accepted. In the summer of 1970, Arna and I loaded the kids into our two cars, a Dodge Dart and a station wagon, and drove to Boston. I thought I was done with basic research forever, but I couldn't have been more wrong.

SIX

Breaking the Rules at Mass General

The patient was crashing. He was slipping into shock after a surgery that had seemed to go fine. I was in the early days of my residency at Mass General, embedded with a surgical team and charged with treating patients after surgeries. The subject in front of me was not doing well: blood pressure plummeting, kidneys shutting down, consciousness coming and going. Several members of the house staff had taken a look at him and gone over his numbers, but nobody could figure out what was wrong. Mystified by the sudden downturn in vital signs, I approached the patient's bedside to chat with him and assess the situation.

I took his hand in mine as a gentle greeting and instantaneously had a flash of insight. The man's hand was big and meaty. During my time at the NIH, I had seen dozens of patients whose hands were big and meaty in exactly the same way. All of these patients had acromegaly, which meant they had tumors of the pituitary gland that were secreting large amounts of growth hormone, leading to enlarged hands. Such tumors also resulted in altered facial features, which I realized this subject also possessed, and impaired secretion of other pituitary hormones that are necessary for the body to respond properly to stress, such as the stress of having just undergone surgery.

"I'm 90 percent certain this patient has acromegaly," I declared to the other hospital staff when I stepped out of the room. "We need to get him on prednisone right away."

The prednisone treatment improved the patient's condition almost immediately.[1] He ended up making a complete recovery, and subsequent tests revealed that he did in fact have a pituitary tumor, which was later removed. I had only been a resident for two weeks, but instantly became a Mass General legend for diagnosing a difficult case just by shaking the patient's hand. Of course, it was dumb luck: my ability to solve this case was purely serendipitous, due to my exposure to dozens of acromegalic patients at the NIH, but nonetheless my colleagues marveled at my medical abilities as though I had just performed a magic trick.

It felt good to be back on the wards and seeing patients. Everything was going according to the plan I had mapped out with my father in our last conversation, right before his fatal heart attack. I felt at peace with giving up research and getting back to life as a physician.

I also felt at peace in my personal life. Arna and I had moved into a beautiful house in Natick, just outside of Boston.[2] The neighborhood was predominantly Catholic and very friendly. With our three children, we had *by far* the lowest number of children on the block. The McGivillrays across the street had seven children. The house next to them had nine. Two houses down from that was a family with eleven kids. Our small brood notwithstanding, we were accepted into the neighborhood, and the McGivillrays even brought us a cake the day after we moved in. Life was good.

The tranquility of my home life stood in stark contrast to the high drama I often experienced at work. After my first rotation with the surgical team, my next rotation was in the ER. Despite my two years at the NIH, I was still quite young for a resident. I was twenty-seven years old but looked twenty-two, so I was often mistaken for a medical student. When ER patients were unhappy with me, they would often yell, *"I want to see the doctor in charge!"*

"You're looking at him!" I would triumphantly proclaim, trying my best to project confidence. More often than not, I would be challenged like this right in the middle of dealing with chaotic emergencies, which were plentiful in the ER: there is no better place to experience high drama on a daily basis than a hospital emergency room.

One especially dramatic evening began when I was at home, watching a telethon on TV while getting ready to come into the ER. The most famous newscaster in the Boston area was talking to the camera and imploring viewers to donate money. I turned off the TV and drove to work. Right at the start of my shift, an ambulance screeched in with a patient in full cardiac arrest. It was the famous newscaster, who I had just been watching on TV less than an hour earlier. My team and I hustled the newscaster to a table.

The anesthesiology resident who normally performed intubations was not available at that moment, so I had to do it myself. The first try did not go well, and I looked around nervously to see if the anesthesiology resident had responded yet to my page. There was no sign of him, so I gave it a second try and fortunately was able to establish a secure airway. The newscaster was in ventricular fibrillation and one of the nurses was charging up the defibrillator.

"Clear!" I yelled, putting the paddles to the patient's chest. His body lurched, but his heart did not restart.

After a few moments, I shocked him a second time: still nothing. Every ER resuscitation is an adrenaline rush, but this one felt especially intense because of my familiarity with this newscaster: I watched him on TV every night, so I felt like I was trying to revive a dying family member.

Finally, on the third shock, the newscaster's heart leapt back into action. I felt an overwhelming sense of relief and sighed deeply as I heard the persistent ping of his heartbeat beeping on the EKG monitor. The newscaster made a full recovery in the hospital, but I was busy with other patients and never had the chance to meet him when he was conscious. Several weeks later, I watched the newscaster on TV again, delivering the nightly news and looking good as new. I felt proud to have helped save the guy's life; it was the sort of thing I had fantasized about when I was younger and yearning to become a doctor.

I was living my childhood dream, enjoying the clinical work and loving my interactions with the patients, yet at the same time I was beginning to feel vaguely dissatisfied. I realized that I missed research. I missed the stimulation of trying to do something that nobody had ever done before. I missed the into-the-wild-blue-yonder feeling of improvising experiments on the fly and going where the data took me, which is the essence of research. Clinical medicine is the polar opposite of research in this regard: in medicine, you typically try to follow the standard operating procedure. The goal is not to do something creative, but rather to follow established protocols for helping patients. In this way, you enhance patient outcomes and also protect yourself (and the hospital) from being sued for malpractice. However, the cautious approach that is necessary for practicing good medicine can sometimes feel constraining, especially compared to the boundary-pushing adventures of basic research. As a clinician, you hear the same stories of received wisdom over and over again; as a scientist, you have the opportunity to start writing your own stories.

I was experiencing creative urges that were very surprising to me. For most of my time at the NIH, I had been miserable and only wanted to get back to clinical medicine. Now that I was back in the clinic, I could think only about research. It was an epiphany for me to catch myself daydreaming about experiments I wanted to perform. I had several elective rotations coming up as I entered the second half of my residency year at Mass General, and I began wondering if I might be able to use some of that elective time to squeeze in a little research.

I had a clandestine meeting with Edgar Haber to discuss research possibilities. Haber was the chief of the Cardiology Division at Mass General and an accomplished researcher who had worked at the NIH with Nobel Laureate Christian Anfinsen. He had a sizable research lab and told me that he would be happy to give me a lab bench so that I could do some experiments. He and I both understood that this arrangement was against the rules: I was being paid from hospital income, not a research fellowship, so I was supposed to be doing my clinical electives and seeing patients. However, I really wanted to do some research, and Haber really wanted an extra pair of hands in his lab, especially from someone with my pedigree of having published papers with Roth and Pastan at the NIH.

Despite the fact that research was forbidden, I began sneaking into Haber's lab and conducting experiments. Soon I was spending almost all my time in the lab. Haber wanted me to work on a steroid hormone called aldosterone, but I wanted to work on something more closely related to cardiology. My father had died from heart disease; I saw myself as avenging his death by performing cardiology research that might save the lives of cardiac patients in the future. To get started, I tried some experiments measuring glucagon binding to cardiac tissue, but rapidly became frustrated by the lack of tools available to target the glucagon system. Next, I switched my focus to the hormone that exerts perhaps the most dramatic effects of all on the heart: adrenaline.

◆

When something scary happens, like if you're hiking and suddenly a bear ambles out onto the path in front of you, adrenaline is released from your adrenal glands into your bloodstream. This hormone mediates the "fight-or-flight" response and exerts particularly striking effects on the heart, which begins pumping harder and faster to get blood out to the skeletal muscles to facilitate fighting or fleeing. In the early 1970s, the only thing known about how adrenaline worked was that it raised cyclic AMP levels inside cardiac cells. It was speculated that there must be a receptor for adrenaline in cardiac tissue, but nothing at all was known about the properties of this hypothetical receptor.

In addition to having a connection to cardiology, adrenaline was attractive to me for another reason: chemical tools had recently been developed targeting the adrenaline system. Specifically, a class of drugs had been created in the late 1960s to block the action of adrenaline at the hypothetical "beta" receptors mediating the rises in cyclic AMP. These so-called "beta blockers" were now being given to cardiac patients around the world to prevent adrenaline from overstimulating their hearts. From the research perspective, I viewed beta blockers not just as drugs for enhancing cardiac health, but also as important tools that could be used to study adrenaline receptors.

I created a labeled version of noradrenaline (a close relative of adrenaline) and began studying its binding to cardiac tissue.[3] To make sure I was studying noradrenaline binding sites that were relevant to the clinical action of beta blockers, I assessed whether my noradrenaline binding was blocked by beta blockers. At first, progress was quite slow, but eventually I figured out the right conditions to measure robust binding of noradrenaline to heart tissue. I became convinced that I was on the verge of making a big discovery and perhaps becoming the first person to identify the beta subtype of adrenaline receptor (also known as the "beta-adrenergic receptor") at the molecular level.

One evening, while I was surreptitiously working late in the lab, disaster struck: I got busted by the house staff director, Dan Federman. He was taking an unusual route through the building because it was raining, and happened to walk right by my laboratory as I was crossing the hallway while carrying a rack of test tubes.

"Lefkowitz! What the hell are you doing here?" he demanded. "I heard rumors that you were doing research . . . You know that's not allowed! See me in my office at 9:00 A.M. tomorrow."

I tried to protest, but no words came out of my mouth. There was no point in arguing anyway: I had been caught conducting research in flagrante delicto. Federman had nabbed me walking out of a research lab wearing a lab coat and carrying test tubes, which is about as red-handed as you can get caught. I went home and told Arna that I might be dismissed from the Mass General residency program. When I went to bed, I couldn't sleep at all. I tossed and turned and kept chastising myself over and over. How could I be so stupid? I had jeopardized my entire career. And for what? Just to do a few experiments?

When morning came, I went to Federman's office with bloodshot eyes and a churning feeling in the pit of my stomach. Federman was sitting at his desk. Next to him was Alex Leaf, the chair of the Department of Medicine. *This is bad,* I thought to myself. *This is exactly how they would boot somebody out of the program.* Federman spoke first and got right to the point.

"Lefkowitz, for the past six months, you were supposed to be doing your sub-specialty rotations: nephrology, dermatology, endocrine, et cetera. Instead, you've blown off every single one of your rotations to spend your time playing with test tubes in the lab, even though you are well aware that taking time out of the clinic for research is completely against the rules."

He paused and glared at me.

"What do you have to say for yourself?"

I launched into a rambling answer about how I felt I needed to get back to research, and also how I thought it might not matter much if I skipped my electives because I knew I wanted to do cardiology. I begged them not to blame Haber for giving me a lab bench, as Haber had undoubtedly assumed I would just squeeze in a few experiments between shifts rather than working full-time in the lab. As I was finishing, Leaf's lips were creasing into a smirk.

"Tell me about your research," he said. "It sounds interesting."

I was momentarily tongue-tied, as I had not expected such a query. It made sense, though, as Leaf himself was an accomplished researcher in renal physiology. When he expressed curiosity about my work, I suddenly began to feel better about the situation. After a brief pause to gather my thoughts, I began to explain my research, my voice rising with enthusiasm as I shared some recent findings I found especially exciting. Federman seemed completely unmoved, but Leaf looked engaged as he peppered me with several questions. Finally, Federman broke up our discussion.

"Dr. Leaf, what should we do with this fellow?"

"Well, it's too late in the game to start a clinical elective now," Leaf said to me. "You may as well just finish up your research for the next few weeks before you begin your cardiology fellowship. But . . . do *not* tell anyone that you skipped an elective to do research. We don't want any of the other residents getting any funny ideas."

I exhaled deeply when I left the meeting. I had been worrying my career might be over, but somehow I had lived to do research another day. You'd think this near-death experience would've scared me straight and caused me to clean up my act. As it turned out, though, my behavior only got more rebellious as I finished up my residency and began my fellowship in cardiology.

◆

Moonlighting was strictly forbidden for all residents and house staff at Mass General. Despite this ban, I held *three* different moonlighting jobs during my time in Boston. I was making peanuts as a resident, and Arna had just given birth to our daughter Mara. Now with four young children to support, plus a big mortgage on our new house, I was under extreme financial pressure. I was on the prowl for whatever moonlighting gigs might be available, despite the prohibition on such positions.

My first moonlighting job was doing insurance physicals. An insurance company would give me the names of clients, and I would drive to their houses and do in-home physicals so that they could buy insurance. The problem with this job was that I was too good at it. I would find heart murmurs in lots of patients, and I even diagnosed one guy with a cancer he didn't know he had. Such diagnoses, however, were the last thing the insurance agents wanted to hear. They wanted to sell the patients insurance, not find health issues that would make the patients ineligible for insurance policies. After one exam, I got a call from one of the agents.

"You marked this guy down as having a grade-two heart murmur," the agent said. "He's not going to be able to get insurance with that."

"I'm sorry," I replied. "But the guy's heart has a murmur."

"Look, I've heard from some of the other agents that you've caused trouble in the past," the agent continued. "If you're not willing to rewrite this guy's exam, I'm afraid we won't be able to hire you again."

Clearly, my reputation for being too rigorous was getting around, and eventually I stopped receiving calls to do insurance physicals. This job only paid fifteen dollars per physical anyway, and it was time consuming because of all the driving around town, so I wasn't sad to see it end.

My second moonlighting job paid much better. After working a full day at Mass General, I would occasionally work a twelve-hour night shift in the ER at Cambridge City Hospital across town and get paid two hundred and fifty dollars, which seemed like a fortune. One time, I was working a late-night shift in Cambridge when one of my closest friends, Bob Gibson, came in as a patient. Bob was my frequent running partner as well as a fellow resident at Mass General, so I was surprised to see him at Cambridge City.

"Bob, what you are doing here?" I asked. "Why didn't you go to the General?"

"Well, I knew that you were moonlighting here tonight," Bob said with a wan smile, looking quite ill. "And there's nobody in the world I'd rather have take care of me than you."

Bob had a hacking cough and high fever, and I rapidly diagnosed him with pneumonia. I got him started on the appropriate antibiotics and set him up in an overnight room because I wanted to keep an eye on him. I was distressed to see my friend in such rough shape, but also honored that he sought me out at Cambridge City to care for him rather than going to our home base at Mass General. It was nice to know that my peers considered me a doctor's doctor, which truly is the highest praise a physician can receive.

My third moonlighting job during my time at Mass General was the most lucrative and also the most interesting. It started when a guy walked into the Mass General ER during my rotation there and filled out a form saying that he didn't want to talk to a nurse but needed instead to see the doctor privately. Such requests usually indicated a patient with venereal disease or some other embarrassing condition. I met the patient in the exam room and asked what was up.

"Well, doc, I'm actually not here because I'm sick," he said. "I'm the Revere High School football coach, and we're required to have a physician at all our games. I'm looking to hire somebody. We pay a hundred and fifty dollars per game, and the physician just needs to sit on the bench and check out any injuries that occur. Do you think there's anyone on the house staff that might be interested in this position?"

"You're looking at him," I proclaimed.

For the next three years, I spent a dozen Saturday afternoons each autumn as the team doctor for the Revere High School football team. My young sons, David and Larry, would usually come with me and sit on the bench. They loved watching the games and hanging out with the players. I mostly just sat on the bench too, although a few times per game a player would go down with a serious injury, and I'd jog out onto the field. Fortunately, I would be accompanied by the team's very knowledgeable trainer, which was good because I was not experienced in orthopedics. We'd look at the player who was down and have a similar conversation almost every time.

"Well, what do you think, Gus?" I would ask.

"I think his shoulder's dislocated," the trainer would answer as the player writhed in pain with a limp arm.

"And what do you think we should do for that?" I'd inquire.

"Pop it back into the joint," Gus would say confidently.

"Do you want to take the first shot?" I'd ask. Gus would then yank on the kid's arm, there would be a loud popping sound and suddenly the kid would be able to move his arm again.

There were sometimes more dire medical issues. One time, somebody in the stands had a heart attack during a game. Another time, a fan had a grand mal seizure. Owing to my ER training, I was actually much more comfortable dealing with emergency situations like these than dealing with run-of-the-mill football injuries. Most of the time, though, there wasn't much to do, so it was good money for light work. Moreover, the coach, Silvio Cella, was a character and I loved seeing him in action.[4] Revere was the worst team in the league, losing many of their games by sizable margins. At halftime of most games, they would already be down by two or three touchdowns, and Coach Cella would give the same speech in the locker room.

"You guys are pathetic. Without a doubt, that was some of the worst football I have ever seen. You're an embarrassment to our school and an embarrassment to the town of Revere. I am disgusted by what I just saw." The players would be hanging their heads. Coach Cella would pace around and continue.

"Everybody out there is laughing at you. Any reasonable coach would just give up on you right now. But you know what: *not me*. I still believe in you. I see the good things you do in practice, and I know you can play better. In fact, if we pull together right now, if we stand united like brothers and play as a team, I believe we can still win this game."

Every week, after breaking the players down and telling them how terrible they were, the coach would build them back up until they were completely pumped for the second half. He'd have them jumping around and bumping chests and breathing fire. Then they'd run back onto the field for the second half and get creamed again. However, the coach was clearly connecting with his players, and the team's losses were not for lack of inspiration. I took mental notes about the coach's psychological tricks for motivating his troops. Many years later, I would use some of these same methods when I was directing my own laboratory and needed to get my trainees fired up during a rough patch in their research.

◆

Despite the time I was dedicating to my moonlighting jobs, and despite the intensity of my training in cardiology, I still continued to sneak into the research lab whenever possible during my cardiology fellowship. I was absolutely in love with research. My experiments felt like forays into a magical world filled with mysterious realms that I was the first to explore. My fellow cardiology trainees appreciated my passion for research and sometimes even covered for me so that I could spend more time in the lab. On several occasions, I would be in the lab doing experiments when a code was called, which meant a patient was in full cardiac arrest, and I would have to drop my test tubes and race over to the clinic to resuscitate a dying patient. Saving the lives of heart attack patients was my job, but research had become my passion.

My mentor Edgar Haber was excited by my research progress and began making efforts to keep me around. He made arrangements for Harvard to offer me the position of instructor, the lowest rung on the faculty ladder, when my cardiology fellowship ended. He also arranged research space for me. There was an old supply closet near his lab that had been cleared out and reconfigured with two short research benches. In this tiny closet-turned-lab, there was just enough room for me and one other slender person to work back-to-back. It wasn't much, but it was a space to call my own.

A few days later, as I was finishing up cardiology rounds, I received a surprising phone call. The voice on the other end was Andy Wallace, the chief of Cardiology at the Duke University Medical Center. He said that he was starting a new program in "molecular cardiology," a phrase I had never heard before, and he wanted me to come give a talk at Duke to interview for a position. I had never met Wallace, but he said that he had seen me present my data at the American Heart Association meeting in each of the past two years and was an admirer. He thought my research was exciting and perfect for the program he had in mind, which would be focused on studying the heart at the molecular level. I had zero interest in leaving Mass General, but figured it was nice to be invited to give a research seminar. Without giving it much thought, I told him, *"Sure, why not, I'll come for a visit."*

SEVEN

"Duke? I Never Heard of It."

My plane was coming in for landing at the Raleigh-Durham Airport and I was worried. Down below, on the airport grounds, not a single other plane was in sight. I had just come from Logan Airport in Boston, where hundreds of planes were tooling around the airport, so it was disconcerting to be landing on a barren runway with no other aircraft in view. After the plane landed, I walked inside the tiny terminal looking for a baggage carousel, but realized there wasn't one. Instead, the baggage from the plane came flinging out of a chute on the exterior of the building and was dumped directly onto the street. This was my first impression of North Carolina.

Despite my initial concerns, my visit to Duke was enjoyable. I gave two talks about my research: a grand rounds presentation to the Department of Medicine and a seminar to the Department of Biochemistry. I met with Andy Wallace and also his boss, Jim Wyngaarden, the chair of Medicine. I stayed at the Carolina Inn in Chapel Hill; when I inquired why I couldn't stay closer to campus, I was told there were no suitable hotels in Durham. As I was heading back to the airport, I informed my taxi driver that I was flying Eastern Airlines, and he laughed out loud.

"There are only two gates, my friend, so it doesn't really matter what airline you're flying!"

Shortly after I returned to the hustle and bustle of Boston, a priority mail letter arrived with a job offer from Duke. The offer was for an appointment as an assistant professor in the Department of Medicine and a joint appointment in the Department of Biochemistry. The salary was $27,000, which was robust for a junior faculty member in 1973 and significantly more than what I would be making as an instructor at Harvard. The offer also included start-up funds to outfit my lab, which would consist of 1,000 square feet of bench space in the brand-new Sands Building.

I replied immediately to thank Wallace and Wyndaarden but also tell them that I had already committed to staying at Mass General and Harvard. My refusal of their offer prompted a phone call from Wallace.

"Bob, we really want you to come to Duke. What would it take to get you here?" I told him I just wasn't sure, so he said, "Well, why don't you think about it. Go ahead and send me a detailed letter stating exactly what it would take for you to come join the faculty at Duke."

I was dead set against moving to North Carolina, but wasn't sure how to convey this fact. I figured the best way to get Wallace to stop bothering me would be to send him a list of demands that was too preposterous to be met. I thought about it for a few days and put together the craziest list of demands I could dream up. Instead of 1,000 square feet of lab space, which was already ten times the size of my closet-turned-lab at Mass General, I asked for 1,500 square feet. In addition to the sizable start-up funds Duke was already offering, I insisted that I would also need guaranteed salary for both a technician for three years *and* a postdoctoral fellow for three years. Finally, I demanded to be appointed as associate professor with tenure. This ultimatum was especially outrageous given that I was not yet even a faculty member at Harvard. For someone who is not yet a faculty member to demand tenure is beyond brash, but I was trying to be over the top on purpose. They wanted demands, so I gave them.

After I sent Wallace the letter, several weeks passed and I figured I would never hear from Duke again. Then one day on cardiology rounds, someone yelled that there was a phone call for me. I picked up the receiver and Wallace was on the line.

"Congratulations, Bob! You're coming to Duke!"

"What do you mean?" I asked, dumbfounded.

"We met your demands!" Wallace continued. When I asked which ones, he bellowed, "All of them!"

I was stunned. I asked Wallace to give me a few days to wrap my head around this development. The first thing I did was go home and talk to Arna. She understood the mind-blowing nature of the offer from Duke and told me that I would be crazy not to take it. She pointed out that I was literally working in a closet at Mass General, but at Duke I could have a real lab as well as a huge amount of money to launch the research program I was envisioning. Arna was also game to experience living in the South, and painted the move as a big adventure for us and the kids.

Next, I set up a meeting to talk with Alex Leaf, the chair of Medicine at Mass General. I wasn't expecting a counteroffer, but simply felt it was a professional courtesy for me to discuss Duke's offer with him. To my surprise, Leaf requested twenty-four hours to come up with a counteroffer.

The next day, I walked back into Leaf's office and his face was beaming with a proud smile.

"Bob, we have a deal worked out, and we think you're going to like it," he said. "Next year, instead of becoming instructor, we're going to make you chief medical resident. Then, after that, you'll become an instructor."

My jaw dropped. This was the best counteroffer that Mass General and Harvard could muster? I knew that serving as chief medical resident at Mass General was a tremendous honor that could open a lot of doors for someone in a clinically focused career. However, I also knew that the position of chief resident was a 24/7 job that would not allow any opportunity for me to conduct research. My heart was telling me to spend *more* time doing research, not less, so this counteroffer, though on the surface enticing, was completely out of step with how I was feeling.

I tried to hide my disappointment from Leaf and told him I would think about it. The next day, I informed him that I had accepted the offer from Duke.

◆

Arna and I visited our family in New York to tell them about our impending move to North Carolina. The news did not go over well. My mother gasped and immediately began kvetching about how far away her grandchildren would be. Arna's mother was flat-out dismissive.

"Duke? I never heard of it," she scoffed. "Is it new?"

I informed her that Duke had been around for many years and was considered an up-and-coming university, but she was not impressed. She had heard of Harvard and could understand why her son-in-law might want to stay in Boston to take a faculty job at the most famous university in the world. However, she could not understand why her son-in-law would want to move her daughter and grandchildren hundreds of miles away to take a job at some unknown school in what seemed to her like the middle of nowhere. I may as well have told her that we were moving to the tip of South America.

When the time came for us to move, Arna and I packed up our belongings into our two cars and began the journey from Boston to Durham. The kids were split up between the cars, with two in each vehicle. However, it was the summer of 1973, and I was obsessed with listening to John Dean's testimony in the Watergate hearings. Dean was being interviewed by the Senate eight hours each day, and his descriptions of President Nixon's wrongdoings were absolutely riveting. In my car, the only thing on the radio was the Watergate hearings. In contrast, Arna was playing Top 40 music, so the kids decided that driving with Mom was more fun. Halfway through our journey, we ended up moving most of the luggage into my car to create space for the kids to ride with Arna.

Upon arriving in Durham, we promptly got lost. We stopped to ask a woman for directions, and she pointed us toward Hillsborough Road and said it would be the third traffic light. Shortly after pulling away, I noticed a car speeding up behind us: it was the woman who had just given us directions, and she was frantically waving her arms. She pulled alongside of us, rolling her windows down and speaking breathlessly.

"I know I told y'all that Hillsborough was the third traffic light, but then I realized it's actually the fourth traffic light. Sorry about that! I just want to make sure y'all get there in good shape."

We thanked her and drove off. After we arrived at our house, I marveled to Arna about how nice the woman had been in giving us directions. In New York City you would be hard-pressed to find a person who was even willing to stop to give you directions, never mind someone who would chase you down afterward to correct themselves and apologize if the directions weren't perfect. This was my first taste of Southern hospitality, and it increased my confidence that we had made the right choice in moving south.

We began setting up our new house, and meanwhile at work I began setting up my new lab. I had given the Duke administrators a list of equipment to order, and all of this equipment was now sitting in boxes in my gigantic lab space. Fortunately, I was not alone, as I had brought with me a technician named Fritzie Erlenmeyer from Mass General. I had worked with Fritzie in Haber's lab and thought she was terrific. She was an unmarried woman in her sixties with no family obligations keeping her in Boston, so we worked out a deal where she would accompany me as a temporary technician for three months to help me set up my new lab at Duke. She knew how to assemble all the equipment and perform all the assays, so she could help train a new technician and also train any postdoctoral fellows or students who joined the lab. She was absolutely invaluable to me in my first few months in North Carolina.

With a huge amount of empty lab space that needed to be filled, I started bringing in other personnel to join the lab. My hiring strategy was simple: take anyone who walked in the door. Prior to my move, Andy Wallace had informed me that he had met a young scientist named Lee Limbird who was just finishing her Ph.D. at the University of North Carolina in Chapel Hill. She wanted to stay in the area because her husband was doing a residency at Duke, and her interests seemed aligned with mine. I told Wallace to go ahead and hire her on my behalf, even though I had never met her.

There was a guy named Marc Caron who had written to me when I was still in Boston and he was finishing his Ph.D. at the University of Miami. He was mistakenly under the impression that I had my own group at Harvard, even though I was actually just a cardiology fellow working as part of Haber's group. I did nothing at the time to disabuse him of his misconception. Caron told me he was a Canadian citizen and could probably get a postdoctoral fellowship from Canada to pay his salary. That sounded great, I told him, and by the way I had just accepted an offer from Duke so I would be moving soon. Caron said that was fine and shortly thereafter he received his Canadian fellowship, so I hired him sight unseen to join me at Duke.

A third person who joined my group at Duke was a young M.D./Ph.D. student named Rusty Williams. He wandered into my office on July 1, 1973, which I remember because it was the first official day of my employment. Rusty was as skinny as a rail and spoke with a strong Southern accent. He said that he was looking for a lab to join to start his Ph.D. studies and was interested in my research. I knew nothing about this kid and hadn't seen his transcripts or any letters of recommendation. However, he seemed bright and I needed some warm bodies in my lab, so I said sure, he could join.

As fate would have it, all three of my initial hires would go on to become superstar scientists. Lee Limbird would become a standout professor at Vanderbilt and eventually chair of the Department of Pharmacology and then become provost. Marc Caron would end up staying at Duke, launching his own lab, becoming a James B. Duke Professor (the highest honor bestowed by the university on faculty), and winning numerous prizes for his research in pharmacology and neuroscience. Rusty Williams would go on to become professor at the University of California at San Francisco, be elected to the National Academy of Sciences, and found two thriving companies in the Bay Area.

I have no idea how my first three hires all achieved such stratospheric levels of success. I would love to claim credit (and often do) for being an amazing judge of talent, but the reality is that at this early point in my career I was simply accepting anybody who applied. I hadn't even met two of these three hires, and the third was a kid who literally just wandered in off the street. Was it luck? Was it destiny? I have pondered this question for a long time without finding an answer. All I can say for sure is that seemingly overnight, my empty lab at Duke was suddenly filled with a bunch of bright young minds who brought incredible energy and enthusiasm to the space.

The lab's first year was marked by youthful exuberance and intensity. Lee set the tone with her hyperkinetic personality. She worked at a manic pace, and in between experiments she would perform miniature workouts in the lab. Her favorite mini-workouts were "bicycle rides," where she would lay on the floor, prop her hips up in the air, and spin her legs as if riding a bicycle. One time, I was hosting a visit from a distinguished Yale professor and wanted to show off my new lab. As we walked through the lab door, the first thing he saw was a pair of female legs spinning furiously in the air. The Yale professor turned to me with a bemused look on his face.

"What kind of operation are you running here, Bob?"

It was my job to channel my lab's youthful enthusiasm into productive directions. I was a mentor now. I didn't have any experience mentoring during my time at the NIH or Mass General, as I had just been focused on doing my own experiments. All of a sudden, though, I was required to offer direction to all these young scientists who had joined my group. In growing into the role of mentor, I made more than a few mistakes. For example, one day I saw that Rusty had centrifuged some tissue extracts and was preparing to separate the solid membrane pellets from the liquid supernatants (or "soups"). Sensing that my young student needed assistance and feeling confident in my own bench skills, I strode over and snatched the centrifuge tubes from Rusty's hands, eager to show him the proper technique. I took the tubes over to the sink and went into a dramatic crouch, elbows akimbo.

"Okay, Rusty, watch carefully. You gotta get your elbows out, then snap your wrist at a ninety-degree angle," I said as I poured the soups off into the sink and down the drain. "Then snap the wrist back up to avoid disturbing the pellet." I proudly showed him the intact pellets, but then noticed that Rusty's eyes had widened in horror.

"Yes, I see," said Rusty. "But for this experiment, I don't want the pellets. I wanted the soups!"

As a new investigator, I also made mistakes in handling my lab's budget. Like most new medical school professors, I had zero training in budget management and hadn't spent much time at all thinking about the cost of research equipment or reagents. The size of my group at Duke was growing rapidly and we were ordering whatever we wanted without keeping careful track of our spending, so it was not long before we significantly overspent the lab's research budget. I received a stern call from the Department of Medicine business manager, an intimidating former

Marine named Jim Mau. He read me the riot act for having overspent my lab's budget by more than $50,000, a huge sum at that time. Mau threatened to shut my laboratory down, and for several days I was worried sick that I would be forced to tell all my enthusiastic young students and postdocs that we had to close up shop for a while. Thankfully, my boss, Jim Wyngaarden, stepped in and said that he would cover the overdraft using the department's discretionary funds. I thanked Jim profusely and vowed to do a better job in keeping track of my lab's spending.

I also made rookie mistakes when it came to regulatory affairs. We were trying to improve on the radioligand binding assays I had performed at Mass General, and one idea we had was to label the beta-adrenergic receptors with radioactive beta blockers rather than radioactive noradrenaline. Beta blockers were known to bind more tightly to beta receptors than noradrenaline did, and our hope was that the beta blockers would therefore be superior tools for labeling the receptors. Marc Caron and I asked a company called New England Nuclear to create a radiolabeled version of an obscure beta blocker known as alprenolol, the chemical structure of which suggested that it would be relatively straightforward to label with radioactive tritium. In our order, though, we didn't specify how much radioactive material should be shipped to us.

After a few weeks, when the radiolabeled alprenolol arrived from New England Nuclear, we received a panicked phone call from the Duke radiation safety officer. The amount of radioactive tritium in the sample was 1.2 curies, which was more than was allowed in the entire state of North Carolina! Quick phone calls were made to state regulators to get a special dispensation to use this level of radioactivity, and fortunately everything was approved and we were not tossed in jail for breaking state law.

Using the radiolabeled beta blocker, Marc and I achieved incredible results in just a few months. The alprenolol binding to tissue samples was highly specific, and the pharmacological profile of the binding sites demonstrated that we were indeed labeling authentic beta-adrenergic receptors. Lee and Rusty joined in to help extend this work, as did two new postdocs who had just joined the lab, Wayne Alexander and Chabirani "Chobi" Mukherjee. As a group we were excited by the alprenolol binding data and debated whether we should show these findings at a big international meeting in Vancouver, Canada, in the summer of 1974. Having heard rumors of competition, we decided to keep the data to ourselves and not talk about this work at the meeting. As soon as we got to the conference, though, we immediately learned that *two* other groups had the same idea to use radiolabeled beta blockers to label beta receptors, and these groups were both presenting their findings at the meeting.[1] It was obvious that the race was on. So we changed our plan and began telling everyone who would listen about our exciting new data, as we wanted the world to know that we were also in the race. This generated a lot of buzz, and when we returned to Duke we immediately wrote up our data and then rapidly published a series of papers reporting the use of tritiated alprenolol to label beta receptors.[2]

It was exhilarating to be racing against top scientists from around the world to publish our data. For the first time, I began having a grand vision of where this research might lead. At the meeting in Vancouver, I recall sitting on the bed in my hotel room, with Lee, Marc, and Rusty gathered around, and expressing my ambitious view as to where we were headed. I enthused to the members of my lab about how the simple binding assay we had developed for the beta receptor might be leveraged to make rapid advances. For example, we could become the first group to study whether there were changes in the numbers of beta receptors in different disease states or following certain drug treatments. Even more importantly, we could at last prove the existence of the hypothetical receptors that had been controversial for decades, purify these receptors, learn their molecular identity, and eventually try to unravel their three-dimensional structure. I was no longer satisfied to just indirectly study the properties of receptors; I wanted to directly interrogate them, know all their secrets, and take them apart and put them back together again like a mechanic dissecting a car's engine. I felt a swelling sense of excitement that my lab could be the first to take all these steps and lead a revolution in understanding what receptors are and how they work.

We returned to Duke from the meeting in Vancouver fired up and ready to go. It wasn't long, though, before I was back at the airport and off on another trip. I was starting to get numerous invitations to speak at conferences around the country, as well as requests to serve in leadership roles for national societies. I had never been much of a world traveler in my younger days, but now I was becoming a regular at the Raleigh-Durham Airport, which fortunately was undergoing a major expansion: they even had baggage carousels now, so my bags no longer had to get thrown to the pavement at the end of each trip. Just a few years after I arrived at Duke, I found myself regularly jetting around the world to talk about my research and experiencing one adventure after another.

EIGHT

Travelin' Man

I was sitting in the copilot seat of a plane that was headed straight for the side of a mountain. My mind raced with thoughts of my soon-to-be-fatherless children.

In my fifth year as a faculty member at Duke, I was elected by my fellow members of the American Federation for Clinical Research (AFCR) to serve on the AFCR Council. After my election, I was excited to learn that my first council meeting would be held on the small island of Tortola in the British Virgin Islands. To get there, I flew into Puerto Rico and then took a single-propeller puddle jumper to Tortola, which had an airport consisting of a single runway and one small building that looked like a mobile home.

When the council meeting was over, the small group of us who were serving on the council headed back to the tiny airport. When we arrived, it was pouring rain and not a single soul was in sight. There *was* a single-propeller plane sitting on the runway, but nobody was around to fly it.

We waited for over an hour, and then finally a guy drove up, got out of his pickup truck, and climbed into the plane. He spent a few minutes trying to start the plane without success, then got out and banged on the propeller a few times. When he got back in the cockpit, the plane finally started and several puffs of black smoke emanated from the engine. The group of us who were waiting began to look at each other in consternation, wondering if this was supposed to be our ride.

The pilot taxied down the runway and took off without us. The plane barely cleared a mountain that was close to the runway and then headed out to sea. We all breathed a collective sigh of relief that this piece of junk was not our aircraft. Moments later, though, the plane looped around over the water and came back in for a landing. The pilot got out, came over to the mobile home where we were waiting and said, *"Okay, is everyone ready to go?"*

"Are you sure that plane is okay?" one of my colleagues asked. "It seemed like it was hard for you to get it started."

"Oh yeah," the pilot said. "It gets a little balky sometimes, but I got it up in the air and everything seems okay."

Before we boarded, everyone had to be weighed so that the load could be evenly distributed on the plane. My weight turned out to be identical to that of the pilot, so I had the honor of sitting next to him in the copilot's seat. As the pilot flipped a bunch of switches and prepared for takeoff, I looked him over: he had a big bushy mustache, wore a pair of bandoliers in an "X" across his chest, and had an unlit but well-chewed cigar dangling from his mouth. He struggled to start the plane again but eventually got it going and began trundling down the runway through the rain and wind.

Once we were airborne, the plane was once again headed straight for the mountain. The pilot was fighting the wind and trying to gain altitude, and for a solid minute it looked as though we were going to pancake right into the mountainside. At the last second, though, the plane gained enough altitude and we crested the mountain by a few feet. My knuckles were white and my heart nearly stopped, but at least now we were over open water. With some time to get my bearings in the tiny cockpit, I surveyed the instruments and noted that the fuel gauge was squarely on E.

"Excuse me, is this the fuel gauge?" I asked. When the pilot nodded yes, I said, "Well, I'm not an expert, but it looks like it's reading empty."

The pilot reached over and flicked the fuel gauge a few times with his finger. Each time he flicked it, the gauge bounced around between E and quarter-full, and then settled back to empty.

"Don't worry about it," the pilot said. "I think we have enough fuel. This gauge hasn't been working for a while now."

The pilot's words did not exactly inspire me with confidence. I felt the urge to tell my travel companions in the seats behind me about our questionable fuel situation, but at the same time I didn't want to alarm them. Moreover, even if we had concerns about the pilot's judgment, there wasn't much we could do at this point in the trip. What were our options? Hijack the plane and turn back to Tortola? I kept silent but was bursting with anxiety for most of the flight until the lights of Puerto Rico came into view. We landed without incident and I felt like kissing the ground when we got out of the plane.

Travel is a constant in the lifestyle of a modern researcher. It's not enough to just conduct experiments and publish papers—it's also necessary to attend scientific meetings to present your findings to others. These meetings are where collaborations are established, reputations are made, and careers are developed. Moreover, as a scientist's reputation grows, it is also expected that they will take leadership roles in *organizing* scientific meetings, which is what I was doing in Tortola as part of the AFCR Council. In addition to attending and organizing meetings, many scientists also consult for drug companies to help with the translation of basic research findings into new therapeutics. Starting in the late 1970s,

I began serving as a consultant for several different companies, with each of these jobs requiring extensive travel. I spent a lot of time crossing time zones, which wreaked havoc on my body clock.

On one occasion, I flew to New York to receive a research prize and then flew directly to London to consult for the pharmaceutical company SmithKline. I was functioning on almost no sleep and spent a full day advising the company, then had just a few hours to catch up on sleep before flying back home to the USA. I was worried that I wouldn't be able to sleep due to jet lag, so I took two Halcion tablets to help me get to sleep quickly at the hotel in London. I snuggled into my comfortable hotel bed and fell into a deep slumber.

When I woke up, I was on an airplane. I had absolutely no idea how I got there. I looked out the window and saw that the plane was high over the ocean. Confused, I turned to the guy next to me.

"Excuse me," I asked sheepishly. "This may sound like a strange question, but can you please tell me what flight I'm on?"

The guy looked at me like I was crazy. "Yeah, uh, this is Flight 644 and we're headed to JFK Airport in New York. We're about halfway there."

"Okay, thanks," I said. "Again, this is going to sound weird, but have I been acting oddly?"

"Not really," the guy said. "You got yourself settled, put your bag away and you've been asleep ever since."

I had heard that sleepwalking could be a potential side effect of Halcion.[1] But had I really sleepwalked, or perhaps somehow "sleep traveled" via unknown conveyance, all the way from my hotel room through London to Heathrow Airport? And if so, what kind of shape was I in?

I got up from my seat and headed to the bathroom. To my surprise, I found that I was neatly groomed: my face was clean-shaven and my clothes looked normal. I returned to my seat and looked through my carry-on bag, finding all of my items in their usual places. Somehow, it appeared that I had carried out several different complex tasks, including dressing, packing, and navigating an airport, but had absolutely no memory of any of it. It was one of the most shocking experiences of my life.

A few years after this incident occurred, I told the story to my friend Jerry Olefsky, a distinguished researcher at the University of California San Diego. His response was, *"I can top that."*

"No way," I said.

Jerry proceeded to tell me a story about the time he took a drug similar to Halcion to help him get some sleep while traveling, and then he suddenly woke up at a reception. He was holding a drink and standing in front of a colleague whom he had known for many years.

"Excuse me, this is very embarrassing," Jerry said to his colleague. "Can you tell me what's going on here?"

"Are you alright, Jerry?" his colleague asked in a concerned tone.

"I'm not sure," said Jerry. "Please tell me what's going on."

"Well," said the colleague. "You just gave your lecture, and now we're at the reception."

Jerry was stunned. "How was my lecture?"

"It was great," his colleague said. "Just like always."

"Were there questions?" asked Jerry.

"Yeah, of course," replied his colleague. "There was a question and answer session, and you answered everything they threw at you."

I had to admit that as amazing as my story of having lost all memory of getting to the airport and boarding a plane was, Jerry's drug-induced inability to remember having just given an entire lecture (and taken questions) was even more amazing.

❖

As my career progressed, I became a more experienced traveler. In later years, I would often mix in sightseeing with work-related travel, but as a young gun trying to establish my reputation, I was only thinking about work. Sometimes this intense level of focus got me into trouble. For instance, at one scientific meeting held in downtown San Francisco, not far from the so-called Tenderloin District, I took a break from the meeting to have lunch at a local deli. While eating, I pored over the program booklet, checking off the talks in the various sessions that I would try to hear. As I hurried back to the meeting, I found myself walking in step with a young woman in a smartly tailored business suit, heading in the same direction. I smiled at her, and after a few pleasantries she asked, *"What do you like this afternoon?"*

I pointed out several interesting talks that had caught my eye. *"No, no,"* she responded, *"What would you like to do?"* I wasn't sure how to respond but murmured something about maybe trying the trolley if the program wasn't so packed. With mounting exasperation, she gave it one last try, explaining directly that she was not attending the meeting but was in fact a hooker looking for clients. Feeling embarrassed that I had been too dense to catch her meaning, I thanked her and graciously declined, going on to explain that I would be busy chairing the afternoon cardiovascular session.

While some scientific meetings are held in major cities like San Francisco, many research meetings are held in more rustic venues where there is a strong emphasis on roughing it. For instance, the prestigious Gordon Research Conferences were held for many years almost exclusively in the summertime at private residential high schools in rural New England. With the students away for the summer, the student dorm rooms served as lodging for the scientists who attended the meetings. These rooms were tiny and had no air conditioning. I never cared much for these spartan accommodations, and typically tried to at least finagle my own room in order to get a little more space.

At one Gordon Research Conference in the 1970s, I showed up late to the meeting and asked about getting my own room, but was told it was impossible. The woman checking me in said the meeting was fully booked, so the best she could do was to put me in a room with another scientist who currently had a double room to himself. She gave me my room number and noted that the meeting was currently on afternoon break for several hours, so I had time to go to my room and get settled in before the evening session. I walked up several flights of stairs on a sweltering hot New Hampshire day and finally made it to my room. The door was ajar, so I knocked gently and walked in. As I entered the room, my nostrils stung with the smell of intense body odor. I had a sudden impulse to avert my eyes and flee; instead, I soldiered on and was aghast by what I saw.

Lying buck naked on one of the beds was a large, hairy man who was perspiring heavily and snoring. He was fast asleep, with two large flies circling lazily around his head and occasionally landing on him. The stench in the room was as foul as anything I have smelled in my entire life, including cadavers in medical school. I stood inside the doorway with my suitcase at my side, trying to decide what to do. I thought to myself: *Am I really going to room with this creature?*

I stepped back outside into the hallway, quietly closing the door behind me. I then went back downstairs to the woman running the registration desk, walked up to her and made a matter-of-fact statement.

"I'm sorry, but I can't sleep in that room."

"Why not?" she asked. I explained the situation—the large hairy man, the foul stench, the flies—and she was sympathetic. However, she also said that there were no other rooms available.

"I don't care," I said. "I'll sleep on the floor somewhere if I have to. But I'm not going back there."

"Okay, Dr. Lefkowitz, I have another idea," she said in a hushed, conspiratorial tone. "I'm not supposed to do this, but we do have a couple of beds in the infirmary in case anyone gets sick. Nobody is in there right now, so you can have one of those beds if you like."

I gratefully accepted her offer and headed to the infirmary. I wasn't sure what to expect, but compared to the tiny dorm rooms, the infirmary was positively luxurious. There was a ton of space, the beds were adjustable in the style of hospital beds, and rather than sharing a bathroom with a dozen other people, the infirmary had its own bathroom. In subsequent Gordon Conferences that were overcrowded, I would use this trick again on multiple occasions, asking to sleep in the infirmary in order to secure more spacious accommodations for the week.

At this time, Gordon Conferences were viewed as the gold standard of scientific meetings with the power to make or break young scientists' reputations. At my first Gordon Conference, which was focused on molecular pharmacology and held in the mid-1970s, I felt like a total outsider. The meeting was dominated by disciples of the legendary Nobel Laureate Earl Sutherland, who had passed away a short time earlier. The Sutherland gang—Al Gilman, Joel Hardman, Al Robison, and others—were all now faculty members at elite research schools and ranked among the biggest names in the field. They sat in the back of the room and ran the meeting like it was *The Gong Show*: if they didn't like a talk, they would begin jeering and hooting and cackling. Everybody in the audience kept one eye on the speaker and one eye on the Sutherland guys to see what their reaction would be. After noting this dynamic on the first day of the meeting, I felt intimidated the next day before giving my own talk, but did my best to block out the crowd's reaction and just focus on telling my story.

One of the few people I did know at this meeting was Lutz Birnbaumer, who had worked down the hall from me during my Yellow Beret days. Lutz was now a faculty member at Baylor, and, like the Sutherland gang, was considered scientific royalty at these meetings because he had worked at the NIH with the revered Marty Rodbell. In contrast, I was a nobody. Yes, I had published a couple of decent papers with Roth and Pastan, but Jesse and Ira were endocrinologists, not hardcore pharmacology researchers like the crowd at these Gordon Conferences. Given my lack of pedigree, I worked diligently at these meetings to give sharp presentations, ask incisive questions following other talks, and schmooze with other researchers during lunch and coffee breaks in order to learn what made them tick.

After several years of regular attendance at these meetings, I felt like I was beginning to gain the respect of my peers, if not necessarily their friendship. One summer in the early 1980s, Gilman, Birnbaumer, and I were all invited to speak at three distinct Gordon Conferences. The meetings were held during the same ten-day period and located within fifty miles of each other, so it would've been reasonable for Gilman, Birnbaumer, and I to carpool between the meetings to save on transportation costs and share some company. At this time, though, there was a lot of competition between our labs and emotions were running high, so we ended up just driving our own individual rental cars between the meetings like some sort of passive-aggressive convoy. In truth, I never could have shared a car with Gilman in any case because he smoked like a chimney. During outdoor coffee-break discussions at Gordon Conferences, I always stood upwind of Al, because standing downwind guaranteed an eye-watering cloud of secondhand smoke and a jolt of nicotine that could paralyze a moose.

My travel schedule grew more grueling with each passing year. These efforts were worth it, though, as my service in scientific societies, consultant jobs for various companies, and attendance at conferences helped cement my reputation as an up-and-coming researcher. I began to build relationships with other scientific leaders and understand them as individuals, as opposed to just knowing their names from reading published papers. These new connections, in turn, led to new career opportunities. Temptation was knocking, and I needed to decide how I was going to answer.

NINE

Learning to Say No

The dean of the Duke University Medical Center, Bill Anlyan, called me in for a meeting, saying he had an important matter to discuss. I had no idea what to expect. I waited outside his office, wondering if I was in trouble. Finally, Anlyan called me inside and got right down to business.

"Bob, the chairman of the Department of Pharmacology is retiring, so we need a new chair. I believe you'd be terrific in the position. What do you think?"

I was thirty-three years old and had been at Duke for a little more than three years. I was flattered to be considered for such a leadership position, and aware that the job would come with a substantial salary increase. However, this position would also come with extensive administrative responsibilities that would be a major drain on my time. The politically correct response would've been for me to tell Anlyan I would think about it, but instead a truthful answer just came spilling out of me.

"Well, thank you for the consideration, but in all honesty that's not where my heart is right now. My lab is on a roll. We have incredible momentum, and all I want is to focus on keeping that momentum going."

I surprised myself with the speed and force of my answer. You never really know how you're going to react to a shocking offer until it happens, and in this instance the answer just popped out before I had a chance to stop it. Dean Anlyan said he was disappointed, but he understood. I left his office and headed straight back to the lab.

My research program was moving at breakneck speed, and I had begun to feel like a rider on a runaway horse. I didn't know whether I was leading the horse or the horse was leading me; I was just holding onto the horse's neck and trying not to get thrown off. It was exhilarating, and I wanted more of it. What I definitely did *not* want was to get bogged down in all the mundane tasks and daily minutiae that would be associated with running a department. I just wanted to keep riding the horse to see where the adventure would take me next.

During this period, after I had received a couple of big research grants and my research program was fully established at Duke, offers from other schools started to become a normal occurrence, and I had to master the art of politely saying no. A speaking engagement at the University of Iowa afforded me an extended training session in this area. I had been invited to Iowa by their distinguished chairman of Medicine, Francois (Frank) Abboud. At dinner after my seminar, Frank told me that he was founding a new research center at Iowa and wanted me to take the position of chief of the Cardiology Division in his department. Without hesitation, I told him no.

After some unsuccessful arm twisting, the conversation drifted to other matters. Some time later, though, Frank returned again to the issue of recruiting me to Iowa. "You know, Bob, I also need a new chief of the Endocrine Division. Given your endocrinology training at the NIH, you'd be a great fit for that position too. What do you think?"

I told him no again, but he persisted. While our plates were cleared away and we had after-dinner coffee, Frank came back with yet another idea.

"Did I mention that we're starting a new Division of Clinical Pharmacology? You would be the perfect guy to be the *founding* director of this division. We can put together a recruitment package that would be incredible."

I demurred a third time and he threw his arms up in the air.

"Bob, I've offered you chief of Cardiology, chief of Endocrinology, and chief of Clinical Pharmacology. What *do* you want to be chief of?"

"I don't want to be chief of anything!" I laughed. "I appreciate the offers, and I love the programs you're building here in Iowa, but really I just want to focus on my research."

A fundamental key to professional success is knowing when you're in a good situation. At Duke my situation was amazing, and I knew it. I had strong support from my boss, Jim Wyngaarden, and other campus leaders. Wyngaarden had my back when I had overspent my lab's budget during my first year, and I felt deeply that he and other leaders at Duke were committed to helping me achieve success. Even more importantly, I had a growing lab filled with talented young scientists. We were on an incredible journey into uncharted terrain in a very competitive field. I didn't know exactly where we were going, but it was exciting, and I knew we had to move quickly. If I had taken an offer from another school at that point, it would've taken me months to move the lab and get things set up again in another location. With all the lost time from the move, we would've fallen behind the other groups who were on our heels. My instincts were telling me to stay at Duke and just keep powering forward rather than worry about fancy titles or how much money I was making.

To efficiently deal with the deluge of offers I was receiving from other schools, I composed three different generic letters turning down such requests. These three letters conveyed varying levels of angst, with the amount of angst being proportional to the stature of the university.

Letter C was polite and brief. Letter B was longer and indicated a higher level of angst. Letter A was reserved for inquiries from the top universities in the country. I would wait a week, conveying that I was agonizing over the decision, then send a letter saying:

"I am honored to be considered for this position at your prestigious institution. It truly made my day to receive your invitation, and I am humbled to even be considered. I've spent the past week discussing the matter with my family, and I wish I was able to proceed forward in more serious conversations with you. However, for a variety of personal reasons, I'm afraid that I am not in a position to be considered further at this time. Thank you again for the honor you have bestowed on me with this invitation."

The key to politely declining professional offers is to cite personal reasons. If you cite a professional reason for wanting to stay in your current position, it sounds like you're negotiating. For example, if you mention that you don't want to leave your current position because you are happy with your large amount of lab space, this will only incite other schools to say that they can offer even more space. However, if you cite personal reasons, this shuts the door to any future attempts at negotiation. Furthermore, it's important that the personal reasons be unspecified; if you mention something specific, like your spouse doesn't want to move because of their job, another school may take this as a cue to hire a headhunter to help your spouse find a new position in their area. Thus, even though my primary reason for not wanting to leave Duke was that I didn't want to lose momentum in my lab's research, I always cited unspecified personal reasons when declining recruitment offers from other schools. And in a way, I was telling the truth. My lab was personal to me—I had put my heart and soul into the research we were conducting and didn't want to do anything to jeopardize it. So "personal reasons" it was.

Many young scientists in the early stages of their independent careers get distracted by constantly chasing the Bigger Better Deal. I have always subscribed to the simple idea that if it ain't broke, don't fix it. I was happy at Duke and enjoying a lot of success, so I didn't want to waste any time or energy getting into discussions with other universities. Along these lines, I also tried to streamline other aspects of my professional life to ensure that I could remain as focused as possible on my research.

The hardest activities for me to give up were my clinical duties. When I first came to Duke, I spent roughly 60 percent of my time on research and 40 percent of my time seeing patients. However, as my research program took off, this ratio rapidly shifted to 70/30, then 80/20, and then 90/10 after a few years. Psychologically, it was difficult for me to reduce my clinical work, as I felt like I had promised my father in our final conversation before his death that I would remain focused on being a physician. In winding down my clinical work and ramping up my research, I felt like I was going back on the promise I had made to my father. However, I also remembered my discussion with my mentor Jesse Roth, when Jesse told me it was impossible to achieve greatness as a researcher, clinician, and administrator. According to Jesse, you had to choose one, and as time wore on, I knew he was right. I chose research.

Every new faculty member, indeed every young professional of any stripe, has to learn to say no. Those who fail to learn this lesson will never achieve the focus that is critical to success. I said no to promotions at Duke. I said no to offers from other universities. I greatly reduced my clinical effort, even though I loved seeing patients. A certain level of service is expected from all faculty members, of course, and I certainly did my fair share—for example, serving on the house staff selection committee each year during my first decade at Duke. However, I turned down many other service requests to concentrate on running my lab.

I said no to numerous opportunities during my first few years at Duke in order to stay focused on research. In mid-1976, however, I received a phone call with an offer I couldn't refuse.

TEN

The Howard Hughes Medical Institute

B ob, good news!" the voice crackled on the other end of the phone. My boss, Jim Wyngaarden, continued talking over the noise in the background. "I'm at the airport, coming back from an advisory board meeting at the Howard Hughes Medical Institute. I wanted to let you know that you're going to be a Hughes investigator."

"I am?" I said. "Wow, that *is* good news. Do I need to do anything?"

"Yes," he replied. "Have a research proposal on my desk by Monday morning." As he said these words, my jaw dropped.

"Jim, it's Friday afternoon. You want me to write an entire research proposal in one weekend?"

"Oh, don't worry about it," he said quickly. "Just take your NIH grant, the one that's already funded, and put a different cover page on it. Have it on my desk by Monday. It's a done deal."

That's how I became an investigator of the Howard Hughes Medical Institute (HHMI). At the time, I was only dimly aware that HHMI existed; the institute was nowhere near as famous in 1976 as it is now. These days, HHMI holds regular nationwide competitions marked by rigorous peer review, with only the best of the best scientists getting funded. When a scientist finds out they've been named a Hughes investigator nowadays, the occasion calls for a bottle of champagne and a week of celebration. In contrast, when I received the call from Jim Wyngaarden in the spring of '76, it didn't seem like that big of a deal.

I would soon learn from Wyngaarden how HHMI worked. It was basically like the Mafia. All Hughes investigators were drawn from the top ten medical schools, which were like Mafia families. Each family had a capo, with Wyngaarden being the capo at Duke. Whenever HHMI wanted to appoint a new round of investigators, the capos were asked to put forward the top young researcher at their institution, with the induction of these young guns into the institute analogous to becoming "made men" in the Mafia. The process for becoming a Hughes investigator changed completely (for the better) in the mid-1980s, when HHMI began sending out an open call to all universities and holding a rigorous review process that was run by a blue-ribbon panel. In the 1970s, though, it was a completely different story.[1]

The driving force of HHMI in the 1970s was staying one step ahead of the Internal Revenue Service. The institute had originally been set up in 1953 as a tax shelter by the eccentric billionaire Howard Hughes. To maintain its status as an institute, HHMI needed to spend a certain amount of its assets each year. If HHMI did not spend the stipulated minimum percentage of its assets, its status would be changed from "institute" to "foundation," a distinction with significant tax consequences. In 1976, HHMI was required for tax reasons to spend some additional money, which led to my appointment as an investigator that year.

The main benefit of becoming a Hughes investigator was that the institute completely covered my salary, which was bumped up to $32,000, a tidy sum in those days. I stayed in my same lab space at Duke and was still a Duke faculty member, but HHMI now paid my salary. Most medical school faculty members need to pay their salaries with hospital revenue by performing clinical work. However, faculty who bring in research grants can pay themselves with research dollars, meaning they can spend less time in the clinic. My appointment as a Hughes investigator therefore allowed me to dramatically curtail my clinical duties and spend more time focused on research, which was exactly what I wanted to do. In addition to the salary coverage, I also received from HHMI a research budget of $10,000 per year, which was decent money in those days, but nowhere near the lavish research budgets that contemporary HHMI investigators receive. Hughes research budgets increased substantially over the years, especially in the 1980s, when HHMI again was required to spend additional money for tax reasons.

Another key benefit of my appointment was that Hughes investigators at that time were not allowed to hold leadership roles, such as serving as a chair or dean. The reason for this rule was that HHMI wanted its investigators to be focused on research, not administrative duties. As far as I was concerned, this HHMI restriction was wonderful, as it gave me another reason to say no to the various leadership positions that were being offered to me. I had already declined a number of leadership positions because I simply wanted to focus on research, and holding an HHMI appointment made it even easier for me to decline future recruitment attempts by other universities.

I learned from Wyngaarden that Hughes appointments had to be renewed every five years, and the review process was stringent. You had to submit a written plan expressing your vision for your lab's research during the next five-year period, and on top of that you had to give a talk at the annual HHMI workshop and get grilled by a review panel. All Hughes investigators gave brief presentations at these annual workshops held at HHMI headquarters in Coconut Grove, Florida, but the investigators who were up for their five-year renewals gave longer talks and then got strafed with questions by the review panel members. During my first few workshops, I learned the code of honor amongst the investigators, wherein we all refrained from asking tough questions of our peers who were giving the renewal presentations, fearing we might embarrass them in front of the review panel and jeopardize their chances for renewal.

At the conclusion of the morning sessions at these annual workshops, we would adjourn for lunch while the review panel sequestered themselves in a small room to make their fateful decisions. As lunch ended, Kenny Wright, the administrator of the institute, would come out, find the individual who had given a renewal presentation that morning, put his arm around them, and walk to the back of the room to deliver the news. We'd all watch the body language, trying to sense whether our colleague was getting a thumbs-up or a thumbs-down, and then we'd rush over to either console or congratulate the poor soul.

Kenny Wright was a piece of work. He was a good ole Southern boy who had once served as the chauffeur to Howard Hughes's personal secretary, Nadine Henley. Somehow, he had parlayed that position into running HHMI. Kenny had no scientific background at all, but he was a sharp judge of character. I sat next to him during a number of the HHMI workshops, and he had an uncanny way of predicting who would get renewed and who would not, even though he didn't understand a word of the science. I never figured out how he did that. The other thing I remember about Kenny is that he never called me "Bob" but instead called me "Bobby," the only person who ever did that other than my family.

At my very first workshop, George Thorn, then the institute's director of research, addressed us after dinner. He talked about all the complaining he had heard about the review process and how tough the institute was in terms of retaining investigators. He then offered us some words that were meant to be reassuring.

"I don't know why all of you fellows are so uptight about the reviews. You should know that as long as you're the number-one man in your field, you'll never have a problem with us."

Yes, it was just that simple! All you had to do was be the absolute best in your field, and everything would be fine—no pressure. By the way, Thorn's admonition that we needed to be the "number-one man" in our field was telling, as HHMI in that era was definitely a boys' club. There were fifty or so investigators in the country at that time, and all were male. The dinners at the annual workshops were typically followed by cigar smoking, whiskey drinking, and lewd storytelling, as if HHMI were less a scientific institute than a raunchy after-hours gentlemen's club. As a mentor who has always promoted women in science and trained a large number of standout female scientists, I'm happy to note that HHMI these days strives hard to be egalitarian and supports the research of numerous outstanding women; in fact, the current president of the institute is a woman (Dr. Erin O'Shea). In the 1970s, though, HHMI was an all-male enclave.

The boys' club vibe of the HHMI scientific workshops in that era was reinforced by the constant presence of two enigmatic characters, Chester Davis and Bill Gay, who were HHMI trustees and core members of Howard Hughes's personal inner circle. Davis was an aggressive lawyer who drank, smoked, and cursed with unbridled intensity. If his wild stories were to be believed, he spent half his time raising horses in Virginia and the other half trotting the globe using Howard Hughes's money to fight Communism. He gave the impression of someone you could go to for a recommendation on buying a good bottle of bourbon or hiring a top-notch hit man. In contrast, Gay was a devout Mormon who didn't drink, smoke, or curse at all, but exuded the air of a man who had seen things that had challenged his faith. It would be impossible to find a more mismatched pair than Davis and Gay, yet they were always hanging out together at the HHMI workshops, rubbing shoulders with the scientists.

The last of the old-school HHMI Directors was Don Fredrickson,[2] who took over in the early 1980s. Fredrickson had been the director of the NIH and thus came to the leadership of the institute with powerful credentials. As soon as he arrived, he decided that there was lot of deadwood amongst HHMI investigators, and he set out to personally visit each of the sites around the country in order to evaluate *every* active investigator, not just those who were up for the normal five-year renewals. These sessions resulted in large numbers of Hughes investigators losing their funding. The situation was further complicated by the unusual nature of the institute's "First Lady" at that time, Fredrickson's wife, who deeply involved herself in institute affairs. She would attend our workshops and the various social activities around them down in Coconut Grove and told us all that she was to be referred to as "Madame" and her husband as "The Doctor." I'll never forget the visit that Fredrickson made to review our group at Duke.

About two weeks before the visit, when tension was already starting to run high, I received a call from Madame. She told me that she had heard I was the senior investigator at Duke and she wanted to give me some tips about the Doctor's preferences, so as to make the visit go as smoothly as possible.

"You do want the visit to go smoothly, don't you?" she asked.

"Of course," I replied.

She told me that the Doctor liked tea at 10:00 A.M., and gave details about what types of tea should be available. She also stated that he liked lunch precisely at noon and preferred chicken salad sandwiches on lightly toasted white bread with the crusts removed. She stressed the importance of removing the crusts. I took careful notes and, at the end of the conversation, went immediately to our business office to make sure that all these requests were fulfilled.

Even more remarkable than Madame's requests was the visit itself. Each investigator at Duke had one hour to present their lab's work. We were told that the time should be divided between the investigator himself and two junior people, either students or postdoctoral fellows from the lab. Each group would present privately to the reviewing team. From my lab, I selected Marc Caron, the most experienced member of my group at that time, as Lee Limbird had already taken a faculty position at Vanderbilt. Marc was about to take a faculty position himself at Duke, so he was certainly an experienced hand who I knew could handle pressure. For my other speaker, I chose Rick Cerione, a relatively new postdoc in the lab. Rick was a lanky Italian guy from New Jersey who was performing some interesting studies at that time, and I wanted to showcase his data for the review committee. Rick was scared stiff, though, about the possibility of screwing up and being responsible for the lab losing our Howard Hughes funding. I spent two weeks before the visit reassuring Rick that it was no big deal, which of course I didn't believe myself.

Rick, Marc, and I assembled at our appointed time outside the room where the HHMI reviews were taking place. One of my Duke colleagues was in the room before us, along with two of his trainees, and we could hear them getting grilled by the Hughes reviewers. Rick was starting to sweat.

"Rick, just hang loose," I told him. "Like I've been saying all week, it's no big deal. You're gonna do great."

All of a sudden, the doors to the room flew open and there was a flurry of activity. The postdoctoral fellow from the group before us was being carried out of the room unconscious, with one arm around Kenny Wright, the HHMI Administrator, and one arm around one of the reviewers. The postdoc was out cold and his feet were dragging behind him. Kenny laid the guy down in the hallway and began trying to revive him. Rick grabbed my arm in a panic.

"I thought you said it was no big deal!"

"Look, Rick, I know this postdoc," I tried to assure him. "The guy is always fainting. He faints if you look at him cross-eyed.[3] Don't worry about him, just focus on your presentation."

A couple of minutes later, it was our turn to present to the HHMI reviewers. I started things off with a fifteen-minute overview of the lab's research, describing our efforts to purify beta-adrenergic receptors and functionally reconstitute them in order to study their activity (as described in the next chapter). I then introduced Rick to talk to the committee about his recent work. Rick looked terrible and was visibly shaking as he stepped to the podium. He attempted to speak, but nothing came out of his mouth. Marc grabbed a cup of water and brought it to Rick, who chugged the cup's contents in several gulps. He then tried to speak again and finally managed to force out a few words.

"My tongue feels very big in my mouth," he said.

It was not the most promising start to a research presentation. At least he was speaking, though. Marc brought him another cup of water, and eventually Rick was able to proceed with his talk. When Rick finished, Marc got up and gave a smooth presentation, and we ended up getting renewed.

It was fortunate that we were able to keep our funding intact, because the research in the lab at that time was firing on all cylinders. In fact, we were about to launch into a run of discoveries that would address the central mystery of our field.

ELEVEN

Two Thousand Frogs
a Week

In the 1970s, many people were skeptical that receptors existed. Belief in the existence of receptors was viewed in some quarters as less respectable than belief in the existence of Bigfoot or the Loch Ness Monster. This was true of even some of the most eminent scientists in the field.

At a national meeting in 1973, I presented a talk outlining my belief in receptors as physical entities as well as my aspiration to prove their existence. This talk was followed by a discussion panel featuring the legendary Raymond Ahlquist as a member. Ahlquist was the researcher who, in 1948, first discerned that there were two types of adrenergic receptor, which he termed alpha and beta. He was also an ardent skeptic of the existence of receptors as physical entities. In addressing the question of whether it might be possible to learn more about alpha and beta receptors by purifying them from tissues to study their properties in isolation, Ahlquist had written that such studies would only be worthwhile *"if I was so presumptuous as to believe that alpha and beta receptors really did exist. There are those that think so and even propose to describe their intimate structure. To me they are an abstract concept conceived to explain observed responses of tissues produced by chemicals of various structure."*[1]

Ahlquist's remarks were clearly intended as a dig at me and the handful of other young Turks at the time who were performing ligand binding studies with an eye toward eventually trying to purify receptors. After my presentation at the meeting, Ahlquist publicly questioned whether my goals made any sense and voiced skepticism that receptors actually existed as physical entities. He wasn't being mean about it; Ahlquist was an avuncular fellow who was always very friendly to me. He just did not believe that receptors existed, and was concerned that I was wasting my time trying to study their molecular properties.

Like all true believers, I never wavered in my conviction that receptors had a physical existence and could be purified and studied in isolation. To me, receptors were like locks, and hormones such as adrenaline were akin to keys that fit into the locks to open a door. Locks can be removed from doors and still function as locks; according to this logic, I believed that receptors could be removed from cell membranes and still function as receptors. In the view of Ahlquist and other skeptics, however, receptors were not like locks at all. In fact, they weren't like anything. Rather, they were some mystical "pattern of forces" in the membrane which had no discrete physical reality but somehow allowed a hormone or drug to act.

The first step in trying to prove Ahlquist and the other skeptics wrong was to develop a radioactive binding assay to track receptors; as described in Chapter 7, we achieved this goal in 1974. Next we needed to find a way to purify the receptors from the cell membranes in which they resided.[2] In the mid-1970s, Marc Caron in my lab spearheaded a heroic effort to purify beta receptors. Our preliminary studies showed that beta receptors were made of protein, but only represented about 1 out of 100,000 proteins in the cell membrane of a typical cell. Thus, in order to completely isolate the receptors, we would need to achieve 100,000-fold purification. To facilitate this daunting task, we needed to collect the largest possible amount of purified receptor, and therefore needed to find the best starting material to use.

Adrenaline exerts profound effects on the heart, but the density of beta receptors mediating these effects in cardiac tissue is surprisingly low. There was already some evidence that there were beta-adrenergic receptors in red blood cells from various species, so we measured receptor numbers with our alprenolol binding assay. To our amazement, we found that the density of beta receptors was much higher in red blood cells from amphibians such as frogs than just about any other tissue we examined. We furthermore found that grass frogs had the highest density of receptors in their red blood cells, with bullfrogs and other types of frogs having much less impressive receptor levels.

We also explored blood samples from a number of related creatures that were bigger and might yield larger quantities of blood. For example, we obtained alligator blood from a gator farm in Florida. I loved the idea of using alligator blood as a source material for this epic venture, given that alligators are such fierce creatures, but unfortunately the alligator blood was nowhere near as spectacular as the grass frog blood in terms of beta receptor density. The most shocking result came when we examined red blood cells from the African clawed toad (*Xenopus laevis*) and found that these cells had no beta receptors at all! Clearly, there were some interesting differences in adrenergic physiology between frogs and toads, but these differences were not our focus. We were simply seeking the richest possible source of beta receptors, and we settled on red blood cells from grass frogs.

At this time, I knew nothing at all about frogs. I didn't even know what frogs ate. As we began obtaining massive numbers of frogs to facilitate our receptor purification efforts, we talked to some experts and learned that the best food for frogs in captivity is crickets. Thus, we began obtaining huge numbers of crickets. But then what about feeding the crickets? Fortunately, we ended up going through our crickets fairly quickly, so there was never a need to concern ourselves with buying cricket food.

As we ramped up our purification efforts in the late 1970s, we began routinely ordering two thousand frogs a week. The frogs would arrive from Mexico in large crates and sit in the Duke Medical Center post office for a while. Inevitably, someone from the loading dock would call my office and say, in a Southern drawl, *"Dr. Lefkowitz, you gotta get these frogs outta here because they are stankin' to high heaven!"* I would then go into the lab and announce that I had received word the frogs were stankin' and we needed to go pick them up.

On days when we would harvest the frog blood, we would set up an assembly line. My lab consisted of about a dozen people at that time, and for the assembly line it was all hands on deck: one person would pith the frogs, such that they were killed instantly and painlessly, another person would inject them with saline, and a third person would exsanguinate them to collect the blood. Other folks in the lab would continuously process the blood samples to prepare them for receptor purification. I frankly never liked having to utilize such large numbers of frogs to facilitate these experiments. However, it was a simple reality that the only way for us to isolate beta receptors was to start with fresh material from living creatures, and frog blood just happened to be the richest source of the treasure that we were seeking.

Pouring gigantic quantities of red blood cell extracts over our custom-designed columns, Marc Caron was able to achieve an impressive purification of the beta receptors. To assess the binding activity of each fraction coming off the column, Marc would perform extensive binding assays with radioactive beta blockers, which meant he was working with substantial amounts of radioactivity on a daily basis. During these years, Marc was in his late twenties but looked about sixteen years old, and I used to tell everyone in the lab that his lack of facial hair was due to all the radioactivity exposure.

Marc's baby face occasionally got him into trouble. One Saturday night, several guys from the lab were heading out to a strip club in nearby Raleigh for a birthday celebration. They invited both Marc and me. I politely declined, figuring that I was the boss and should strive to maintain a professional level of distance, but Marc felt that he should attend to celebrate his friend's birthday. However, as a devout Catholic and a sweet, innocent soul, Marc had never been to a strip club in his life. On top of that, he looked like a teenager who was borderline legal to be in the club. Seeing Marc's baby face and sensing his innocent nature, one of the strippers grabbed him from his seat, brought him up on stage, and somehow managed to get his shirt off. She then danced around Marc, twirling his shirt in the air and rubbing it suggestively across her body while Marc turned every possible shade of red. This story was told again and again for several weeks after the incident and became lab lore that lived on through the generations.

Fortunately, Marc survived his strip joint experience and continued purifying receptors at a brisk clip. He was soon joined by others in the lab, including a young student named Jeff Benovic and a postdoc named Rob Shorr. Rob was a smooth talker who used his skills as a con artist to facilitate the purification effort. He would request quotes for various newfangled columns that we might use as additional purification steps. He would then ask the companies to set up their purification columns in our lab for a week as a demonstration. Moreover, he would ask the salesmen performing these demonstrations to run his samples over the columns so that he could see how well they worked. It reminded me of Tom Sawyer convincing his friends to paint the fence for him; Rob would just sit back and let the salesmen run all his samples while he lounged around the lab and watched. We didn't end up buying very many columns, but we did get a lot of samples nicely purified using this approach.

Ultimately, we were able to achieve more than 100,000-fold purification of the beta receptor from the red blood cells of grass frogs.[3] This meant that we could hold small tubes in our hands that contained pure beta receptor. It was thrilling and incredibly gratifying to hold those samples. However, it was also sobering to realize that we never had more than 25–50 micrograms of receptor at any one time even after weeks and weeks of purification (one microgram is one thousandth of a milligram, or about 0.00000004 ounces). We published a series of papers about our purification efforts, and this work made waves in the field.[4] However, there was still one problem: not everyone believed us. Skeptics asked, *"How do you know you've purified the whole receptor?"* They were right: it was possible that we had only purified *part* of the receptor, the portion important for binding to beta blockers and adrenaline. In order to show that we had purified the *whole* receptor, we needed to put our purified receptors into cells that didn't already have beta receptors and show that we could reconstitute full receptor function. In other words, we needed to show that our putative receptors could convert a cell that couldn't respond to adrenaline into one that could. Quite a bit of biochemical alchemy would be necessary to achieve this feat.

Nobody in my lab had experience with the type of "reconstitution" techniques that would be necessary for these studies. Serendipitously, I had just received an application from a postdoctoral fellow named Rick Cerione (mentioned in the previous chapter about the HHMI review that nearly went awry). Rick was coming from a lab where he had performed reconstitution of various enzymes using techniques that seemed perfectly suited for application to our studies with beta receptors. Typically, I never tried to recruit someone to my lab because they knew a particular technique, as I have always believed in the value of simply taking the best young scientists available and then letting them learn whatever they need to know. In this case, though, we needed to move fast, and Cerione seemed like the perfect match for the next step we needed to take. Rick was Italian-American and had played on the basketball team at Rutgers, so when he visited Duke for his interview I took him out to an Italian joint that had photos of Duke basketball legends on the wall. Needless to say, Rick loved it and decided to come to Duke to join my research group.

Working with cells that contained no beta receptors,[5] Rick collaborated with Berta Strulovici in my lab to show that we could add in our purified receptors to confer responses to adrenaline. With these findings, we were now able to convince even hardcore skeptics that we had purified functional beta receptors. We had shown that our isolated beta receptors carried out both of the core functions of a bona fide receptor: binding drugs with appropriate specificity and activating appropriate cellular pathways. We had finally brought these mythical receptors to life. It was like capturing a live Sasquatch and proving once and for all it was real and not just a figment of someone's overactive imagination. Suddenly, nobody was doubting the existence of receptors anymore; instead, people were jumping into this area and competing with us to make the next big discovery.

We learned through the grapevine that we had serious competition in racing to publish our exciting findings from the reconstitution studies. Al Gilman, my chain-smoking nemesis from the Gordon Conferences, had worked with his colleagues at the University of Texas Southwestern Medical School in Dallas to purify cellular factors that were essential for hormone action through beta receptors and other types of receptors. Gilman and his team called these essential factors "G proteins," and a consensus model was emerging as to how adrenaline might exert its effects through the beta receptor: adrenaline, circulating in the bloodstream, would bind to the beta receptor on the exterior surface of the cell, and this would in turn activate a G protein on the cell's interior. The G protein would then stimulate enzymes to mediate the various effects of adrenaline on cell physiology. To test this idea, there was a race among my lab, Gilman's lab, and several other labs around the world to create a hormone-responsive system by reconstituting three components (purified receptor, purified G protein, and purified enzyme) together in artificial membranes that were solely made up of purified lipids.

My lab was adept at purifying receptors, but to compete with Gilman (a future Nobel Laureate for the discovery of G proteins) and his collaborator, Elliott Ross, in this race we needed to collaborate with other scientists who could supply the purified G proteins and enzymes. Thus, we started a collaboration with my former rival Lutz Birnbaumer (now at Baylor), who knew how to purify G proteins, and the brilliant Eva Neer from Harvard, who knew how to purify adenylyl cyclase, the main enzyme downstream of beta receptor activation. We would ultimately show that indeed we could put these three components together in purified lipid vesicles to create a simple system that responded to adrenaline and produced cyclic AMP. It was a satisfying demonstration of how adrenaline worked and also satisfying to reach this important goal more than a year before Gilman and Ross did.[6]

◆

At the same time as these beta receptor purification efforts were unfolding, we had a number of other interesting projects going on in the lab. Our studies on ligand binding to the beta receptor were revealing bizarre differences in the binding curves of agonists (drugs that activate the receptor) versus antagonists (drugs that block receptor activity). I sensed that these observations might be of seminal importance, but lacked the mathematical background to try to model what might be going on and thereby figure out what the medical and pharmaceutical applications could eventually be. A colleague at the NIH recommended I talk with André de Léan, a young French-Canadian scientist with remarkable mathematical skills and an interest in modeling biological phenomena. André and I hit it off and he moved to North Carolina to join my group at Duke. At that time, André had a prominent mustache and was as bald as a billiard ball; when I introduced him around the lab on his first day, I told the other lab members that André's brainpower was so intense it had burned off all his hair.

For the studies that André wanted to pursue, we needed a lot of computing power, and computers were very expensive in those days. Fortunately, right after André arrived at Duke, I received word from the Howard Hughes Medical Institute that they had extra money they needed to spend right away for tax reasons. All HHMI investigators were asked to put in new requests for spending, and I put in a request for $50,000 for a cutting-edge computer for André. It seemed like an insane request, yet it was approved immediately, and when the computer arrived it was imposing: the hard drive was as big as a desk. There was no room for it in the lab, so we had to house it in the computer science building.

In addition to the computer, we also added another mathematical modeler, a Swiss-German scientist named Ernst Bürgisser. He and André sat together each day in their office and argued about mathematical models for the binding data. Every time I walked into their office, they were furiously scribbling mathematical equations on little slips of paper and shouting at each other. They were quite a pair.

Ultimately, we came up with models that explained the various strange features of our binding data.[7] At first, these models were just meant to explain the binding of drugs to the beta receptor, but eventually we and many other groups found wide applicability of these models to understanding the binding properties of other receptors. The papers that we published in this area drew a lot of attention, and I began getting invitations to meetings about mathematical modeling of biological phenomena.

One such meeting was a workshop held in the early 1980s in the Black Forest in Germany. I invited André to attend with me because I wasn't sure I would be able to answer technical questions about some of the mathematics involved in our model. On the day of our flight to Germany, I arrived at the airport early and boarded the flight. I knew that André was chronically late, so I tried not to stress out as the plane filled up with no sign of André. Finally, all the seats were taken except for the one next to me, and an announcement came over the loudspeaker saying that the boarding door was being closed. I had a sinking feeling in the pit of my stomach as I realized that I was now going to have to present the complex mathematical studies all by myself.

Suddenly, just as the plane was about to push away from the gate, there was a loud banging sound on the boarding door. One of the crew members opened the door and André pushed his way through. Apparently André had arrived at the gate and been told that the boarding door was already locked, but he raced past the ticket taker and started pounding on the door. I breathed a huge sigh of relief seeing André's bald head bobbing down the aisle toward the seat next to me. We ended up making waves at the meeting in Germany thanks to André's ability to explain the groundbreaking models he had spearheaded.

My lab's studies in this era were not just focused on beta receptors: we were also making progress in purifying alpha adrenergic receptors.[8] John Regan was leading the charge in purifying the alpha-2 subtype, whereas Fredrik Leeb-Lundberg, Susanna Cotecchia, and John Lomasney were taking the lead in purifying alpha-1 receptors. We also began collaborations with various labs studying other types of receptors beyond the adrenergic receptors. For example, just down the hall from us was the lab of an intense young rheumatologist named Ralph Snyderman. He was interested in studying receptors found on immune cells, and we collaborated to apply my lab's cutting-edge biochemical techniques to the immune receptors that Ralph was interested in.

Ralph and I had a lot in common. We were both Howard Hughes investigators and also had both served as Yellow Berets at the NIH during the Vietnam War years. Like me, Ralph had taken advantage of wearing his commissioned officer's uniform during that era to fly across the country for free. We shared laughs over our somewhat lame attempts to follow military code when we were in uniform. For example, we were always told that when in uniform it was our responsibility to salute if we encountered a superior ranking officer. Personally, this rule always made me uncomfortable, as I had little training in recognizing the rank of other officers and moreover was never really trained in how to salute properly. Ralph told me that one time when he was flying in his uniform, an officer with a highly decorated chest walked past him at the airport, so he leapt up from his chair and snapped off a crisp salute. The other officer returned his salute and stopped to ask Ralph a question.

"What branch of the service are you in?"

"I'm in the Public Health Service," Ralph responded, "How about you?"

"Oh, I'm not in the service at all," the guy replied. "I'm a pilot for Bolivian Airlines."

In addition to bonding over our Yellow Beret "war stories," Ralph and I also connected due to our shared intensity. We were kindred spirits in our passion for research, working long hours and trying to inspire our trainees to do the same. We had a catchphrase that we both enjoyed bellowing in our labs to exhort our troops to give maximum effort: "When disease takes a holiday, then *we'll* take a holiday!" Beyond our shared personal history and research interests, Ralph and I also bonded over our medical training. We both strove to maintain a foot in the clinical world as physician-scientists even though we were intensely focused on our research. I had reduced my clinical duties when I became a Hughes investigator but didn't get out of the clinic entirely. I still loved interacting with patients, so even with my lab racing at full tilt, I did my best to carve out time to spend in the clinics and on the wards. In my mind, I still thought of myself as a physician, and moreover felt that my clinical efforts kept me focused as a researcher on the long-term goal of helping to cure disease. Notably, I continued to make inpatient teaching rounds with house staff and medical students for many years. The number of hours I was able to spend in the hospital dwindled over time, but there was certainly no shortage of drama during my clinical work at Duke.

TWELVE

"Mystery Physician Saves Man's Life"

The car was wrecked, and the guy in the driver's seat was in bad shape. He was unconscious and his head was covered with blood. I could tell from his ashen appearance and thready pulse that his blood pressure was dangerously low, so he was either in shock or close to it. This was a life-threatening situation, and I was the only person on the scene who could possibly provide care.

We were in Monroe, New York, where Arna and I had taken our kids to visit with family. It was a nice break from the intensity of running my lab at Duke, and even nicer that on this particular evening we were able to leave the kids with Arna's parents while we went out alone. On the drive to dinner, though, we had passed by a gruesome car wreck by the side of the road, and as a physician I felt obligated to stop to see if I could offer assistance.

I'd only been on the Duke faculty for a few years at that point and still had great confidence in my clinical abilities, as I wasn't far removed from my residency, when I was practicing medicine every day. Though there have been a number of instances in my personal life when I was called upon to leap into clinical action, this moment by the side of the road in New York was by far the most dramatic.

I heard the siren from the ambulance and was relieved that help was on the way. After the ambulance arrived, however, I developed concerns about leaving the unconscious patient in the care of the two ambulance drivers. Emergency medical technicians in the modern day are highly trained and typically able to provide outstanding care on the spot, but in the 1970s there was much less rigor in the training received by ambulance personnel. I discerned that these two ambulance drivers who had arrived on the scene knew basically nothing about medicine, so I offered to ride in the ambulance with them to the hospital, and asked Arna to follow behind us in our car.

The patient had lost a significant amount of blood, which was causing his blood pressure to crater. While we sped to the local hospital, I started an IV and began administering fluids in an effort to maintain his blood pressure. I also took steps to minimize his bleeding. By the time we reached the hospital, the guy appeared to have stabilized but had not regained consciousness, and I handed my unknown patient off to the ER staff.

Weeks later, after we had returned to North Carolina, Arna's mother sent us a clipping from the Monroe Gazette, her local newspaper. The headline read, MYSTERY PHYSICIAN SAVES MAN'S LIFE ON ROUTE 17. The article detailed how a prominent local citizen had been in a horrific car accident, and then a doctor had appeared out of nowhere and tended to him. This mysterious physician had accompanied the injured man in the ambulance and kept him alive on the long drive to the hospital. Then, like the Lone Ranger, the unknown physician had simply ridden off into the sunset. Arna's mother recognized the details of the story and asked, *"Was this you?"* I confessed that yes, I was indeed the mystery physician, although I asked her not to tell anyone about it. I like to believe that to this day I remain a mythic figure in the greater Monroe area, a ghostly healer who materializes at night to help injured motorists.

During my early years at Duke, my skills as a physician were finely honed and I still spent a substantial amount of time in the clinic. I was proud of this fact, as it helped me feel like I was keeping the promise I had made to my father before his death that I would become a practicing physician. In making the transition from Boston, the only real problem I encountered in the clinical realm was that I simply could not understand the speech of many of my patients at Duke. Certain patients who came from rural North Carolina had such strong Southern accents that it seemed almost like they were speaking a foreign language—especially to a born-and-bred New Yorker. In a number of clinical rounds early in my Duke career, I would take patient histories and ask questions like *"Have you experienced any irregular heartbeats?"* and the patients would respond by saying what sounded to my ear like *"Nodzer nozah."* I would just nod, even though I had no idea what they were saying. After several days of this, I finally pulled aside one of the interns who was a North Carolina native and asked what phrase the patients were saying that sounded like *"Nodzer nozah."*

"They're saying, 'Not that I know of'," the intern replied.

Despite the language barrier I had to overcome, I still managed to crack a few tough cases. One time, I was finishing up rounds on the medical service with a group of students and house staff when I noted that several beds away there was a patient with a scrum of attending physicians and house staff gathered around. Out of curiosity, I poked my head into the group and saw that the team was from the dermatology division. They were examining a man whose arm had a garish two-inch-long skin lesion, which was elevated, deep red in color and exuding pus.

The team seemed puzzled, and for some reason I decided to immediately chime in.

"Looks like blasto to me."

My snap judgment was that this was a case of blastomycosis, a rare fungal infection. Several of the dermatologists around the bed immediately scoffed at my idea, giving me looks suggesting that they didn't appreciate the input of a young cardiologist who spent most of his time in the lab playing with test tubes. My time was limited, so I left the discussion shortly thereafter, but several days later, one of the residents came up to me with an excited look on his face.

"Dr. Lefkowitz, you'll never believe this, but we ran some tests on that dermatology patient, and he did in fact have blasto," he said. The case ended up being presented that week to the entire Duke medical community during grand rounds, with the lead physician giving me a shout-out for correctly diagnosing this unusual case after viewing the patient for all of ten seconds. To this day, I have no idea why my instant reaction was to pronounce it a case of blastomycosis: perhaps I once saw a photo of a similar lesion in a textbook years earlier and the image was filed away somewhere in my subconscious. In any case, this incident reminded me of the time at Mass General when I had diagnosed a patient with acromegaly by simply shaking the patient's hand; in both cases, I had gained stature amongst my peers as a clinical savant who could instantly diagnose even the most obscure disorders. In truth, I had just gotten lucky on both occasions, serving as a fresh pair of eyes and bringing an outsider's perspective that turned out to be useful.

In addition to making clinical rounds at Duke, I also taught both medical students and graduate students. I had no teaching experience at all when I joined the Duke faculty, so my philosophy was simply to bring the same intensity to my teaching that I brought to my research. One time, I was giving a guest lecture in an advanced seminar course and walked into the room right at the top of the hour. I introduced myself and immediately started into an energetic lecture about receptor theory. There were fifteen students in the class and from my first word they were all scribbling furiously in their notebooks, so I was impressed with their level of attentiveness. After five minutes, though, one of the students raised his hand.

"Excuse me, Dr. Lefkowitz, but I think you're in the wrong room. This class is Biochemistry 101 and the students are taking an exam. I know because I'm the proctor."

I stopped dead in my tracks. It dawned on me that this might explain why all the students were writing so furiously. They were writing answers in their exam booklets.

"Why didn't you stop me sooner?" I asked. The proctor offered a sheepish smile.

"Well, I didn't want to interrupt you, because you were so into it!"

It turned out that I was in the right room but the wrong building. I packed up my belongings, walked briskly to the next building over, and began my energetic lecture again from the top.

At Duke, I discovered that I loved to teach. Indeed, I found myself always teaching: in my lab, in the classroom, on rounds, and even when my wife was giving birth. In 1977, Arna was pregnant with our fifth child. I was excited all throughout the pregnancy, as this would be her first delivery that I would be allowed to attend. For our first four children, I was not allowed to be in the delivery room, even though I was a physician. However, the rules in most hospitals changed in the 1970s, and spouses were now allowed to be present for the birth of their children in most cases.

Arna went a few days past her due date, so her contractions were induced with pitocin, a synthetic form of the hormone oxytocin. At that time, it was already known that the actions of oxytocin to increase uterine contractions had all the hallmarks of being mediated by a specific receptor, very similar to adrenaline stimulation of beta-adrenergic receptors. Thus, after Arna was induced with the pitocin and her contractions began to show up on the monitor, I gave an impromptu lecture to the staff in the labor room about receptor-mediated processes and how there must be an oxytocin receptor that was analogous to the beta receptors my lab was trying to identify. Arna rolled her eyes.

"Thank you, professor," she said sarcastically. She was probably wishing that the rules hadn't changed regarding the ban on spouses in the delivery room. Despite her annoyance with my lecturing about receptors, Arna handled the labor like the pro she was by baby number five, and gave birth to a baby boy named Joshua.

◆

Eventually, though, I would spend more and more time in my research lab and less and less time in the clinics and inpatient services. I reached the point where my clinical duties were reduced to six to eight weeks of rounding each year in the Durham Veteran Affairs (VA) Medical Center. Naturally, this led to an erosion of my clinical abilities. Practicing medicine is like anything: the more you do it, the better you get, and when you stop doing it for long stretches then your skills start to fade. This posed a problem for me each year as I would gear up for my rounds at the VA hospital: to lead rounds, you need the respect of the house staff, but it's difficult to command respect when you're not a full-time physician.

My strategy for winning respect from the house staff was a trick I stole from Joe DiMaggio. The legendary Yankees outfielder was renowned throughout his career for his powerful throwing arm, but his arm grew lame in the last few years of his playing career. He learned that his arm was good for only one strong throw per day. After that, his arm hurt so much he could barely lift it. Rather than save his one strong throw for the actual game, though, he would make his big throw each day *before* the game. Right at the end of warm-ups, when he knew the other team was watching, he would uncork a powerful toss from the outfield that would sail on a perfect line to home plate. The crowd would ooh and aah, and members of the opposing team would all make mental notes to never test the great DiMaggio's arm during the game.

In the later years of my clinical career at Duke, I took a page from DiMaggio's playbook each year on the first day of my rounding stint at the VA hospital. One thing I *knew* I was good at was listening to hearts ("auscultation" in medical parlance), so on that first day of rounds I would find a patient with an interesting heart murmur and require all members of the house staff to listen to it. I would then grill them to describe the murmur and explain what it meant: was it indicative of cardiac valve abnormality, or did it indicate a cardiac shunt or other such issue? My hardball questioning was the equivalent of DiMaggio's powerful throw to home plate during warm-ups. The members of the house staff would all make mental notes not to test my knowledge on future rounds, lest they run the risk of getting raked over the coals again. Had they decided to challenge me, I'm not sure I had another long throw in my repertoire at that point.

During these rounding duties at the VA hospital, my main point of emphasis each year would be on drilling the students and house staff members about the importance of taking detailed patient histories. I always felt that establishing rapports with patients and conducting thorough interviews were my greatest strengths as a physician. In diagnosing tough cases, it is crucial to know the patients' stories, as they often contain keys to diagnoses. To cite just one example, my ability during my junior residency to successfully diagnose and treat the actress who was suffering from hypokalemic alkalosis was entirely dependent on my rapport with her and my attention in listening to her story. As the years went on, though, I noted that these listening skills were becoming lost arts in the practice of medicine. By the 1980s, there were so many fancy new lab tests and imaging techniques that most young clinicians became inclined to take only cursory patient histories, instead relying mainly on the technology to guide their diagnoses. However, there are a lot of things that technology can't detect and can only be learned from patient interviews.

One memorable patient at the VA hospital came in reporting vague lung problems, and so a chest X-ray was ordered. On the X-ray, it was impossible to see the guy's left lung because for some reason the entire left side of his chest cavity was opaque. The students and house staff who were involved in this case were mystified and began ordering a slate of expensive and time-consuming further tests. This made the patient concerned, as he naturally wondered why he was being kept in the hospital for such a long time when he only came in reporting mild shortness of breath. As the attending physician, I realized that the patient had only been interviewed in the most cursory manner, so before ordering the additional tests I interviewed the patient myself in front of the house staff. The patient was a farmer, and I explained to him that the main issue was that we couldn't see the left side of his chest. I asked if he had any idea why that might be the case.

"Hmmm . . . well, the only thing I can think of, doc, is that nine months ago I was riding my tractor up a hill, and the tractor flipped over and landed on me. I went to my local hospital and they said I bled into my chest. I felt pretty sick for a while, but then after a few weeks I began to feel better."

It was immediately clear that this information was relevant to the case. Bleeding in the chest cavity (referred to as a "hemothorax"), if not fully evacuated, can lead to fibrosis or scarring of the lining of the lung cavity and restrictions on breathing. This would explain why the guy's chest looked opaque on the X-ray, and also likely explain his breathing issues. I asked the students and house staff who were involved with this patient how this critical detail of the patient's history could have been missed. Did it not seem relevant that this patient's chest had been crushed by a tractor less than a year earlier? The students involved all learned a lesson, and for years afterward I would cite this case as a prime example of the importance of taking careful patient histories.

During the few weeks each year when I was rounding at the VA hospital, I was asked not to plan any travel so that I could make rounds every day. However, my busy schedule of giving lectures and attending research meetings always meant that I was away for at least a few days during that period. Accordingly, I would ask one or another of the junior faculty members in the Department of Medicine who had spent time in my laboratory to cover for me. Someone I relied on quite heavily for many years was John Raymond, who worked in my lab as a nephrology fellow and, amongst other accomplishments, went on to become president and CEO of the Medical College of Wisconsin. John bailed me out on numerous occasions and covered my VA rounds when I needed to travel. However, on one occasion he told me he could not possibly do it.

"I have a grant due in three days, Bob, and there is no way I can spend the next few days rounding for you. I'm very sorry," he said. I wheedled, cajoled, and begged him to reconsider, but he would not be moved.

"Bob, you always taught me that I have to learn to say no," John said. "So I'm just following your advice."

"Yes, John, you need to say no, just not to me!"

In addition to the taste of my own medicine that day, later in my career I had other reminders about the value of saying no when it came to helping patients outside of the hospital setting. In my younger days, I quite often administered care to any sick or injured person I came across, as when I stopped to help the guy in the car wreck in Monroe, New York. As my career progressed, though, I typically demurred from helping random strangers, since I felt that my clinical skills had eroded from lack of use and most patients would be better off getting treatment from a physician whose clinical skills were sharper and more current. However, there were a few occasions even later in my career when I had no choice but to step forward and treat strangers when emergencies arose.

Once, in the mid-1990s, I was flying home from giving a talk in London. The plane had been in the air for about thirty minutes when the captain's voice crackled over the intercom and asked, *"Are there any doctors on board this flight? We have a passenger who is in need of medical care."* At this point in my career, I knew that my clinical chops were waning, so I didn't raise my hand. To be frank, I was hoping desperately there was another physician on the flight who could handle the situation. A few minutes later, though, the captain's voice came on a second time: *"Again, folks, we are in need of a doctor, so please raise your hand if you might be able to provide some medical assistance."* Nobody else was responding, so finally I raised my hand and flagged down a stewardess, who hustled me immediately to the back of the plane.

I was led to a woman who was clearly having a grand mal seizure. Her arms and legs were shaking uncontrollably and her whole body was convulsing. Her terrified husband sat next to her, and I briefly questioned him and learned that she had no history of epilepsy. The woman seemed to be in status epilepticus, a type of sustained seizure that can be life threatening. The standard treatment for status epilepticus is IV infusion of an antiseizure medication to stop the seizure, but obviously we couldn't do that in the air since no medications were available. There was a tiny first aid kit in the back of the plane, and the only useful item I found in it was an oral airway, which I placed in her mouth to prevent the woman from swallowing her tongue and obstructing her own airway. As I tended to the convulsing woman, one of the other stewardesses appeared.

"The captain wants to see you," she said.

We walked quickly to the front of the plane and into the cockpit. I had never been in a jet cockpit before, and found it to be an eye-popping experience, as dozens of gauges and lights flashed everywhere. The pilot was straight out of Central Casting, a rugged guy in a uniform who asked me what was going on. I explained the woman's medical situation. The pilot processed the information and then turned to me with a serious look in his eyes.

"Doc, you're going to have to tell me what to do here. We're approaching Shannon Airport in Ireland. If you think it's necessary, I can land the plane there to get this woman to a hospital. But this is truly our last chance, because it'll be two thousand miles over open ocean before I can land this plane again."

The tension in the air was palpable. I felt like I was in a movie, and possessed absolute clarity about the role I had to play. I locked eyes with the pilot and spoke in the most dramatic tone I could muster.

"Captain, take her down!"

The pilot immediately began flipping a bunch of switches. "Okay, doc, you better get back to your seat and strap in, because this is going to be one hell of a rapid descent."

I strode briskly back to my seat as the captain announced to the main cabin that we would be making an emergency landing. We then began a harrowing descent that felt like we were plummeting straight down toward Ireland. In no time at all, the wheels were screeching on the tarmac, the plane jerked to a stop, the doors flew open and a team of medical personnel came barreling down the aisle with a gurney toward the woman who was having the seizures. After they got her off the plane, I was asked to talk with the medical personnel, and then the captain shook my hand and chatted with me. When I was back in my seat and we were preparing to take off again, the captain made an announcement over the PA system.

"I would like to thank Dr. Robert Lefkowitz from Duke University, who saved the life of that passenger who just left the plane." The whole cabin erupted in applause. I didn't feel like I had actually done very much, so I didn't feel worthy of the ovation. Sometimes as a physician, though, you have to know when a patient needs more than you can give. In this instance, I had recognized that there was literally nothing on the plane to help the patient, so we needed to get her on the ground as soon as possible. Even though my role in this case was minor, I still took satisfaction from making a judgment call that benefited the patient.

Beyond the joy that I have always taken in treating patients, even in cases less dramatic than that airplane, the other main benefit to my clinical work during the Duke years was that it helped greatly in terms of recruiting people to join my research laboratory. Duke is unusual as a medical school in requiring a full year of research by *all* medical students in their third year. At most medical schools, the first two years are dedicated to basic coursework, including anatomy, physiology, and pharmacology, and then the last two years are focused on clinical rotations in the hospital. At Duke, the basic coursework is condensed into a single year, which means that students start their clinical rotations in the second year. The third year is dedicated to research, and then the final year is focused on clinical rotations. This model has been very successful at Duke, and in recent years has been copied by a number of other medical schools. As someone who began my medical career with zero interest in research until I was forced to try it, I can certainly appreciate the value of exposing medical students to research in order to see if they might discover a passion they didn't know they had.

During my teaching of clinical rounds at Duke, whenever I encountered a sharp second-year medical student who asked interesting questions, I would suggest that they consider joining my research group for their upcoming year of research. In this way, dozens of talented medical students ended up doing research in my lab over the years, in many cases making very substantial contributions.

The first two medical students to join my lab were John Mickey, nicknamed "Long John" because of his height, and Kurt Newman, nicknamed "Needle" because he was constantly sticking other members of the lab to draw their blood.[1] Needle Newman worked on alpha-adrenergic receptors on blood platelets, and to obtain starting material for his research he was constantly on the prowl for victims from whom he could extract blood samples. Just about everyone in the lab at that time donated blood toward these studies; even my long-suffering administrative assistant, Donna Addison, bravely sat for visits from Needle Newman on several occasions.

In addition to helping with the recruitment of medical students to my laboratory, my clinical service at Duke also granted me access to clinical fellows who might be interested in research. Unlike the residency program I had joined at Mass General, where I had to conduct research on the sly as if it were a shameful secret, many of the residency programs at Duke included time built in for fellows to pursue research. Over the years, many clinical fellows joined my lab for a year or two of research and made key contributions. In fact, one unassuming clinical fellow who joined my lab in 1984 would go on to become of one of the most important collaborators of my entire career.

THIRTEEN

The Quest for the Holy Grail

B rian Kobilka did not exactly make a forceful first impression
on me. We were chatting in my office, and he was speaking so
softly that I had to lean in to catch his words. It was his first day
as a clinical fellow in my lab, and also the first time I had ever met him.
When he interviewed at Duke in 1983 for a cardiology fellowship, he had
wanted to meet with me, but I was out of town. After he was accepted
into the cardiology fellowship program, he came back for a second visit,
but I happened to be out of town again. Nonetheless, he wrote to me
and asked if he could do the research portion of his fellowship in my
lab, and I said yes, mainly because he already had a fellowship and I
wouldn't have to pay him any salary.

My expectations for Brian were modest. Clinical fellows like him usually just wanted to do their required year or two of research and then get
back to their work as physicians seeing patients. Moreover, Brian knew
nothing about any of the techniques used in my lab. I assigned him to

work with Marc Caron and Jeff Benovic to learn how to purify beta-adrenergic receptors. After he learned the protocol, I thought perhaps he could use the purified receptors to develop antibodies that could recognize the beta receptor and potentially be useful tools in our lab's research.

Brian joined my lab shortly after a postdoc named Cathy Strader had left. Cathy had a solid three-year run in my lab and then accepted a position at Merck, where she got promoted several times right away and was clearly a mover and a shaker. I viewed Cathy's immediate success at Merck as evidence that she possessed certain traits that were of little use to her during her postdoctoral research days but made a major difference in her industrial career. Specifically, she had managerial ability. As a bench researcher, it doesn't matter that much if you know how to manage people; all you're doing is working at the bench generating data. Once you move into a leadership role, though, it matters a *lot* if you know how to manage people. My theory of Cathy's rise at Merck was that she possessed leadership skills that were hidden during her postdoc years but then flowered once she moved to industry.

After Cathy had been at Merck for a little more than a year, she called me one day out of the blue. She knew I was very interested in identifying the gene that coded for the beta-2 adrenergic receptor, and she proposed a collaboration: my lab would provide purified beta receptors, which we were generating in large amounts at that time, and Merck would provide their expertise in molecular biology to help identify the gene encoding the receptor. I expressed interest in the idea, and Cathy put me in touch with Ed Scolnick, the head of research at Merck, to iron out the details of the deal.

The gene encoding the beta receptor was truly the Holy Grail. At that time, we had become skilled at purifying the beta receptor, but we still didn't know anything about its structure. Identifying the gene could show us what the receptor looked like and how it might function. The gene encoding the beta receptor was a stretch of DNA that was found in every cell of our bodies but hidden amongst the vastness of our chromosomes. In the language of the new field of molecular biology, the gene for the beta receptor could be expressed as a sequence of letters (A, C, G, and T), with each letter representing one of the four building blocks of DNA. This string of letters possessed magical properties; if we could decipher the sequence, it had the power to provide the answers we were seeking. For this reason, the gene encoding the beta receptor was the Holy Grail and a lot of people were chasing it.

One of the other groups on the exact same Grail quest was the lab of Elliott Ross at UT Southwestern. We had edged out Ross in the race to show the first complete functional reconstitution of the beta receptor along with G proteins and cyclase (as described in Chapter 11), and now the race was on to find the receptor's gene. We knew we had a sizable head start over Ross's lab and moreover were faster at purifying receptors. However, one day I received a phone call that rattled me. The call was from my former student Rusty Williams, who was now on the faculty at the University of California San Francisco. Rusty had begun a collaboration with a group at Genentech, and through this collaboration had learned that Elliott Ross was working with Genentech's Axel Ullrich to find the gene encoding the beta receptor. This was distressing news to me because Ullrich was one of the world's foremost experts in gene cloning. He had been the first to identify a number of important genes, and now he was collaborating with the formidable Ross to seek the gene encoding the beta receptor.

Meanwhile, progress with our collaborators at Merck was painfully slow. We were sending the Merck team our precious samples of purified beta receptor, which we had cleaved into peptide fragments. The Merck group then tried to figure out DNA sequences that could potentially code for these peptide fragments and design probes that could be used like fishing hooks to cast into DNA "libraries," with the goal of pulling out the right gene. The effort at Merck was being spearheaded by Richard

Dixon, a hotshot gene jockey who had just completed a postdoctoral fellowship at Johns Hopkins with Nobel Laureate Daniel Nathans. He was talented, but not yet very experienced. To assist Dixon, Ed Scolnick brought in Irving Sigal, a more seasoned molecular biologist at Merck who was one of their big guns. So we had two of the top molecular biologists at Merck working on our project, but progress still remained slow.

Brian Kobilka's work in my lab on the receptor antibodies was also showing very little progress. One day, Brian surprised me by saying he wanted to join the effort to identify the gene encoding the beta receptor. Brian knew nothing at all about molecular biology (i.e., the use of recombinant DNA techniques), which was a relatively new field at that time. Moreover, I also knew very little about this area, so I couldn't really train him. I suggested to Brian that if he were interested in contributing to this project, the best strategy would be to visit Merck and learn from Dixon. Brian enthusiastically took me up on the offer, and the team at Merck said it was fine because they could always use an extra pair of hands.

In late 1984, Brian traveled to Merck headquarters, just outside of Philadelphia, and began voraciously learning molecular biology. Brian and his wife, Tong Sun, had two small children at that time, and Brian did not want to be away for too long. Thus, he spent five days at Merck and then traveled back to Durham to spend the weekend with his family. He did the same thing in a subsequent week, working all day long with Dixon in the lab and then reading molecular biology papers all night. After four weeks of this, Brian announced to me that he had learned enough to set up a molecular biology group within my lab at Duke. He presented me with a list of all equipment and reagents we would need, as well as a detailed plan for how we could pursue studies to complement the ongoing efforts at Merck.

I was stunned. I knew that molecular biology was a relatively new field, but still it typically took scientists several years of training in this area to become experts. Brian had reached a remarkable level of competency in just four weeks. I was impressed with what a quick study he was and gave him all the budget he wanted to set up the molecular biology group at Duke. Moreover, I loved the idea of being able to quest for the Grail in our own lab. I found this approach much more satisfying than simply sending our purified beta receptors to Merck and then relying on the Merck team for all the subsequent steps.

Everybody in my lab was excited by the new techniques and approaches that Brian was bringing in. Marc Caron and Jeff Benovic, who had been so central to the purification effort, began enthusiastically learning the procedures from Brian, as did others in the lab. Marc now had his own lab down the hall, but was still collaborating closely with my lab in the effort to identify the gene encoding the beta receptor. Several new trainees in my lab, including a graduate student named Henrik Dohlman and a postdoctoral fellow named Tom Frielle, joined the molecular biology effort, and I also hired Brian's wife, Tong Sun, as a technician. Tong Sun had a master's degree in microbiology and was familiar with some of the molecular biology techniques that Brian would now be using. Moreover, she and Brian worked very well together and were extremely efficient as a unit. In the first half of 1985, my lab went from knowing almost nothing about molecular biology to having a productive team in place that was sharing ideas with the Merck team and pursuing several different approaches in our quest to find the gene encoding the beta receptor.

In the autumn of 1985, I received another distressing call from Rusty Williams. Rusty said he'd heard from his sources at Genentech that the collaboration between Ross and Ullrich had yielded fruit; they had isolated several stretches of DNA (or "clones") that they believed contained the beta receptor gene. All they had to do now was sequence those clones. DNA sequencing in those days was much more challenging than it is today, but nonetheless it seemed clear that Ross and Ullrich were very close to capturing the Grail.

After hanging up the phone from Rusty, I sat at my desk with my head in my hands. How had it come to this? My lab had spent fifteen years, starting from scratch, systematically developing every procedure that would be necessary to purify the receptors and set up the ultimate elucidation of the gene sequence. We had developed radioactive ligands to track the receptors and cutting-edge techniques to purify the receptors. The idea that some other group was now going to beat us in becoming the first to learn what the receptors actually looked like was galling. Adding further salt to this wound was the fact that Ross and colleagues were beating us using all of the procedures that we had developed and published.

I called a meeting of our molecular biology team and told them the dire news. I then went on a frustrated rant, noting that a short time ago we had held a commanding lead over Ross and Ullrich, but now they had come speeding past us and were on the verge of snatching the prize. The situation was distressing, so I asked everyone on the team to think outside the box and come up with some different approaches that might somehow turn things around in the coming days and weeks.

The next day, Brian came in with a list of new ideas. Number three on the list was an idea to screen a type of DNA library that was completely different from the other libraries we had tried to that point. Specifically, Brian proposed to screen a so-called "genomic" library. The gene libraries that we were screening at that time were all made from complementary DNA (or "cDNA"), which means they were all reverse engineered from RNA and thus contained genes at their relative levels of cellular expression. However, as described in an earlier chapter, beta receptors are found at very low levels in most tissues, so Brian was concerned that looking for the beta receptor gene in a cDNA library might be like looking for a needle in a haystack. In contrast, genomic libraries are simply made from total DNA, so all genes are found at roughly equal levels.

Brian's idea made sense to me, but the team at Merck gave us a multitude of reasons why it wouldn't work. The main reason was that the vast majority of genes are not made up of continuous stretches of DNA, but rather are made up of a series of intermittent sequences known as "exons." In between these exons are stretches of "introns," also known as "junk DNA." The Merck team told us that by screening a genomic library, we might find a small portion of our gene of interest, but we also would get a lot of junk DNA, and it would be all but impossible to distinguish the gene from the junk.

Despite these admonitions from our expert collaborators, Brian screened a genomic library anyway and pulled out several clones. The Merck team also pulled out several clones from Brian's genomic library. As we began sequencing these clones, we found evidence that they might contain the *complete* gene encoding the beta-2 adrenergic receptor. Talk about luck! It turned out that the gene encoding the beta receptor was one of just a handful of genes known at the time that did not contain any junk DNA. Thus, screening a genomic library was actually the perfect approach to find this gene, despite the fact that such screens had seemed like an act of naïveté and desperation when Brian had first suggested the idea.

At both Merck and Duke, we began sequencing the clones that seemed to contain the entire sequence of the receptor, and by focusing on different regions of the gene between the two labs we rapidly got most of the gene sequenced. However, there was one problematic stretch of the sequence that Merck was working on and tried to read multiple times, but for some reason just couldn't get a handle on. Our effort stalled out for several weeks, and we spent each day hoping that Ross and Ullrich had also encountered some technical delays in the sequencing of their clones.

During this period, Brian worked around the clock and tried every trick in the book to finish the sequencing. One day, he was immersed in a series of timed sequencing reactions when the fire alarm went off. Everyone in the building had to evacuate, but Brian couldn't leave his sequencing reactions or it would ruin several days' worth of effort. I figured that if Brian couldn't leave, then I couldn't leave—it was the same principle as "the captain must go down with the ship." If Brian was going to risk getting in trouble to stay with his experiment, or perhaps literally risk going up in flames, then I was going to stand by his side to take the heat with him.

The fire alarm kept blaring. Brian stayed focused on his experiment, but I decided I needed to do some scouting to see what was going on. We were several floors up, and I stepped out of a side door onto a walkway to get a view of the fire trucks that had assembled in front of the building. Suddenly, one of the fire marshals spotted me and called me out.

"Hey, you up there! We need *everyone* out of the building! Get out now or I'm coming up there to get you!"

With an adrenaline-fueled burst of speed, I darted back inside the building and sprinted to the lab.

"Brian, the fire marshal just saw me, we have to hide!"

I turned off the lights and moved away from the door while Brian continued processing the samples for his sequencing reaction. I was cursing under my breath about potentially losing several days of work because somebody pulled a fire alarm; meanwhile, Brian was cool as a cucumber, calmly attending to his samples in the semidarkness. I was dying to poke my head out the door to see where the fire marshal was, but I didn't want to get spotted again. After what seemed like an eternity, the fire alarm finally stopped and people began pouring back into the building. Somehow, we had evaded detection and managed to keep the sequencing reaction going.

Brian's sequencing reactions from that dramatic afternoon made progress, and then several days later Brian tried a new approach to finish sequencing the gene's problem region. Using this new approach, he was able to read most of the sequence, and then he set up another sequencing reaction to read the final portion. This second sequencing reaction wouldn't be complete until the evening, and Brian was planning to stay with the reaction and read it as soon as possible. Around 6:00 P.M., I told Brian I was heading home for dinner, but asked him to call me if indeed he was able to read the final stretch of sequence. That evening, I had dinner with Arna and the kids, but was distracted by visions that our quest might finally be at an end.

Slightly past 8:00 P.M., the phone rang. It was Brian, speaking in a calm voice but delivering bombshell news: he now had the final complete sequence of the gene. I called Marc Caron and Jeff Benovic, and the four of us met in the lab around 9:00 P.M. The gene sequence looked good, so I called Merck to share the news. The call was answered by the night watchman, but he was able to put me in touch with Irving Sigal at home. Sigal was ecstatic, and we immediately began plotting our publication strategy.

We knew that we had to move quickly, because we had no idea whether Ross and Ullrich had already completed their gene sequence and submitted it for publication. For all we knew, their manuscript describing the gene sequence was already under review. In those days, there was no Internet, so the fastest way to exchange manuscript drafts for editing was to ship printed copies via FedEx. We began shipping drafts of the manuscript and figures to Strader, Dixon, and Sigal every other day, and they would make edits and then FedEx the manuscript back to us. After several such cycles, we learned that FedEx had just begun offering a "premium" service, which was even faster than their regular shipping. This premium service was rumored to involve a new technology where FedEx could take a document in one city, magically print it in another city, and then deliver a copy of the document the same day. We later learned that this new technology was called a "fax," and it seemed absolutely miraculous to us because we had no idea it was possible to transmit manuscripts so rapidly.

After two weeks of rapid back-and-forth to write the manuscript, we submitted the paper to *Nature*, one of the world's leading scientific journals. The manuscript was reviewed in record time, less than three weeks, and the reviewers had only one major issue for us to address.[1] While we were addressing that issue, the galleys for the manuscript arrived from *Nature*; in an unprecedented maneuver, they were sending us the galleys before the manuscript was even officially accepted. The *Nature* editors were as motivated as we were to get this discovery into press as rapidly as possible, because if another journal were to publish the gene sequence for the beta receptor before us, it would greatly decrease the impact of our *Nature* paper. After we addressed the issue raised by the reviewers, we added the necessary edits directly to the galleys and the manuscript went straight to press.[2]

The *Nature* editors told us that our paper would be published on May 1, 1986. We were forbidden from speaking about our results until that date in order to avoid reducing the impact of the publication, but starting on May 1 we were allowed to discuss the findings in public. As fate would have it, I was scheduled to chair a session at a major scientific meeting about receptors at Cold Spring Harbor in New York on May 1, so I decided this venue would be perfect for the first public unveiling of the beta receptor gene sequence.

Brian Kobilka came with me to the meeting at Cold Spring Harbor, and our hearts sank when we saw the program and realized that Elliott Ross was scheduled to speak right before me. We didn't know for sure whether Ross and his team had the complete sequence for the beta receptor gene. However, if Ross *did* have the sequence, then I sure as hell didn't want him showing it right before I spoke. We had come this far in our quest, and I would be damned if I was going to let Ross steal our thunder at the last minute. I told Brian that I was going to use my prerogative as the chair of the session to switch the order of the speakers. Brian was mortified.

"Can you do that?" he asked in a hushed tone.

"I'm the chair of the session," I intoned in a dramatic voice. "Of course I can do it!"

On the day of the session, I informed the meeting organizers that I was switching the order of the talks because I wanted to open the session with a brief overview of the history of the field. This was true, and indeed I did open up with a historical survey, but of course the main reason for the switch was that I didn't want to risk being upstaged by Ross. I gave my talk and drew gasps and applause from the crowd when I showed the beta receptor gene sequence and discussed some of its surprising features. It turned out it was good that I went first, because right after me Elliott Ross got up and showed a very similar sequence, which had led him and his team to draw many of the same conclusions.

I did feel badly about switching the order of the talks. When it comes to my research, I'm a very competitive person, and in this case perhaps my competitive instincts got the best of me. I was acutely aware, though, that the order of these oral presentations only mattered for that day; what really mattered in the eyes of history would be the dates on which our findings were officially published. After our talks, I congratulated Ross on his findings and asked with trepidation where his work stood with regard to publication.

"Well, we are working on the manuscript and hope to submit fairly soon," he answered.[3] "How about you guys?"

"Our paper is coming out today in *Nature*," I said matter-of-factly. Ross's face dropped. He shook my hand in congratulations, a gentleman as always, but could not hide his disappointment.

When I saw Brian after the session, I shared the news with him: the Grail was ours.

◆

Competitive instincts can become intense when big scientific discoveries are in the offing. Indeed, important scientific breakthroughs are often based on heated competitions between labs, with such races having the salutary effect of speeding up the pace of scientific advances. In our case, we almost certainly would not have moved as quickly as we did in identifying the beta receptor gene if not for the competition from exceptional scientists like Ross, Ullrich, and others. There are many other notable examples of such competitions throughout the history of science, with perhaps the most famous being the race to determine the double helical structure of DNA. This race pitted James Watson and Francis Crick against Linus Pauling, as told with great gusto by Watson in his bestselling book *The Double Helix*. A number of such competitive discoveries have culminated in Nobel Prizes, and in some cases the accompanying antagonisms have become so acrimonious that the participants have not spoken to each other for years afterward. Fortunately, that was not the end result of this particular competition, as I always shared a lot of mutual respect with Elliott Ross, Axel Ullrich, and others involved in the quest to identify the beta receptor gene.

It should be emphasized that the race to understand the nature of receptors was more of a marathon than a sprint. The climactic push to identify the specific sequence of the beta-2 receptor was a finishing kick that lasted for several months, but my colleagues and I had been working toward this goal for more than fifteen years. Two other labs that were part of this long race during the 1970s and 1980s were the labs of J. Craig Venter at the NIH and of Alexander Levitzki at the Hebrew University of Jerusalem. Later on in his career, Venter would achieve fame and fortune as the leader of a private effort to sequence the human genome, which competed with the federally funded Human Genome Project and effectively fought it to a draw. Many years later, in several public talks at which I was present, Venter jokingly credited me with his subsequent success. As he told it, for a period of fifteen years his lab had competed with mine and been scooped by us at every significant point. The cloning of the beta receptor gene was for him the last straw, and he realized he needed to find a different line of work. After losing this race, he became interested in developing technologies to sequence DNA more quickly, and ultimately decided to sequence the human genome. And the rest, as they say, is history.

Similarly, Levitzki also left the adrenergic receptor field after he met with the same fate as Venter. Again, the cloning of the beta receptor gene was apparently the turning point. Levitzki went on to achieve glory in the growth factor receptor field, including the development of many drugs that inhibit growth factor receptor signaling and are widely used in research today. I have often joked that I deserve some measure of credit for the development of these drugs as well as credit for the sequencing of the human genome, since by winning the race against Levitzki and Venter I pushed them out of the adrenergic receptor field and into other pursuits where they achieved greatness. Both men were ultimately elected to the USA National Academy of Sciences, one of the highest honors in science.

FOURTEEN

The Rosetta Stone

T he most amazing thing about finding the Holy Grail was that right before our eyes it magically transformed into the Rosetta Stone.

During the weeks when we were sequencing the gene encoding the beta receptor, word got out on the Duke campus that we were on the verge of a big discovery. Everywhere I went on campus, my colleagues would ask, *"How is the sequencing going? What does the receptor look like?"* My answer was always the same.

"This receptor isn't going to look like anything. It's the first receptor of its type to be identified, so it's going to look completely unique."

As the sequence came into focus, however, I realized that I was spectacularly wrong. The beta-2 adrenergic receptor did look like something else: specifically, it looked like rhodopsin, a light-sensitive protein found in the eye. The primary sequence identity between the beta-2 receptor and rhodopsin was not very high and confined to just one region, but both had seven predicted transmembrane regions and they were clearly related.[1]

I was stunned. Every other person involved in the project—Kobilka, Caron, Strader, Dixon, all the others—was also completely stunned. When I revealed these findings during my talk at Cold Spring Harbor, the audience was stunned. Why would anyone think that the receptor in the heart that responds to adrenaline would look anything like a protein in the eye that responds to light? This shocking revelation had several implications: First, rhodopsin should actually be thought of as a "receptor" for photons of light. Second, if two disparate receptors like rhodopsin and the beta-2 receptor were related in terms of their sequences, then a huge number of other hormone and neurotransmitter receptors must also be closely related. The sequence of the beta-2 receptor was therefore a Rosetta Stone that could be used to decode the sequences of potentially hundreds of other receptors.

After we published our paper with the Merck team in *Nature*, the collaboration with Merck ended. The Merck group was determined to go in their own direction, with a focus on discerning regions of the beta-2 receptor that were important for binding to adrenaline and other ligands. My lab wanted to go in an entirely different direction, with a focus on using the beta-2 receptor as a Rosetta Stone to seek out related receptors in order to test our hypothesis about the existence of a large family of structurally related receptors. Brian Kobilka and others in the lab used the beta-2 receptor sequence to design probes to pull out similar genes.

We assumed that the first DNA sequence that Brian pulled out using the beta-2 receptor sequence must be the beta-1 adrenergic receptor, the receptor most closely related to the beta-2 in terms of function. To our great disappointment, this sequence (which we termed "G-21" as an internal lab moniker) turned out not to code for an adrenergic receptor at all, as the expressed receptor didn't bind well to adrenaline or any other adrenergic ligands. In a serendipitous twist, Tom Frielle, a postdoc in the lab, used the G-21 sequence to pull out a distinct sequence that turned out to be the beta-1 adrenergic receptor.

In parallel, we had ongoing purification efforts in the lab focused on the alpha-adrenergic receptors, as we were seeking to run the table and identify the full set of receptors that respond to adrenaline. These alpha receptor purification efforts were aided by our newly discovered Rosetta Stone. John Regan had been working for years on purifying the alpha-2 adrenergic receptor, with the hope of identifying the receptor's gene sequence. His source was large numbers of platelets from outdated samples of human blood. One of John's early efforts yielded a sequence that didn't look like the beta-2 receptor at all, so we knew it couldn't be right; in fact, this sequence turned out to be derived from HIV, which must have been a contaminant in the blood samples. This was the mid-1980s, before there was any way to screen the blood supply for the AIDS virus. When John told me about this misadventure, he asked for my opinion. I told him my opinion was that he should definitely be wearing gloves while processing these samples.

Eventually, John's persistent efforts led to a breakthrough. Using his purified receptor preparation, he was able to identify a single peptide sequence, which we immediately noted had similarity to a certain region of the beta-2 receptor. This gave us confidence that he actually had the sequence for a receptor this time rather than another virus. Based on this sequence, Brian designed probes, and a short time later pulled out the complete alpha-2 receptor gene sequence. It was dazzling how fast things were moving at this point. All the technical problems that had bedeviled us during our quest for the beta-2 gene sequence had been ironed out, and suddenly it seemed like we were an unstoppable juggernaut that was discovering new receptors at lightning speed.

The other receptor that we had been purifying for years was the alpha-1 adrenergic receptor. Shortly after we identified the gene for the beta-2 receptor, Susanna Cotecchia made a big push to collect enough purified alpha-1 receptor to allow us to hunt for the gene. After nine months of arduous labor, Susanna had collected just enough alpha-1 receptor sample to take one shot at getting peptide sequences. She prepared to load *all* of her precious sample onto a single HPLC column, and several of us stood around her in the lab to offer moral support while she made the fateful injection. Susanna's hand trembled with anxiety as she loaded the sample—if anything went wrong at this point, she could lose nine months of hard work in a matter of seconds. Fortunately, the column ran smoothly. Susanna obtained peptide sequences, and then worked with Brian to design probes to pull out the alpha-1 receptor gene.[2]

Surprisingly, we also discovered a number of receptors we didn't even know existed. At the time, based on functional studies, only four receptors for adrenaline were known: alpha-1, alpha-2, beta-1, and beta-2. Once we started pulling out all the genes, however, we were shocked to find that there were actually three distinct subtypes of alpha-1 receptor, as well as three distinct subtypes of alpha-2 receptor.[3] Altogether, we identified eight subtypes of adrenergic receptor; a group in France then found one more beta receptor subtype (beta-3), which brought the overall number of adrenergic receptors to the unexpected total of nine. As a bonus, we even accidentally identified the first member of what turned out to be a large family of serotonin receptors, as the mysterious "G-21" clone that we pulled out while hunting for the beta-1 receptor was found by Annick Fargin and John Raymond in my lab to be activated by serotonin.[4]

During this heady period, our work was attracting increasing attention, and I wanted to make sure that the young scientists in my lab were receiving appropriate credit for the outstanding work they were doing. In particular, I knew that I needed to promote Brian Kobilka, who was too humble and low-key to promote himself. Around the time of the publication of the *Nature* paper reporting the beta-2 receptor gene sequence, Brian and I attended the annual joint meeting of the American Society for Clinical Investigation (ASCI) and the Association of American Physicians (AAP). Brian had submitted a poster abstract about his work on antibody development, but I told him that he absolutely had to show the beta-2 receptor gene sequence on his poster. Brian protested.

"Nobody will even know that these findings are on my poster, because in the program book my title and abstract say something completely different," he said.

"Leave that to me," I replied.

On the day of Brian's poster, I worked the hall like a carnival barker, drawing sizable crowds and directing them Brian's way. Whenever I saw anyone I knew, I literally grabbed them and brought them over to the poster. When I wasn't grabbing friends and acquaintances, I was working the crowd.

"Come on over to poster board #283! This is a real breakthrough—you do *not* want to miss it!"

Brian was visibly dismayed by my salesmanship. Bodies were five-deep around him, and he was hoarse from shouting to present his poster. It was a trial by fire during Brian's first big national meeting, but it was great exposure for him as a parade of prominent scientists came by to meet him for the first time.

Two years later at the same meeting, I pushed Brian even harder. This time, his abstract was selected (out of thousands of abstracts) to be given as a twelve-minute oral presentation during the plenary session, the biggest session of the meeting. There would be several thousand people in the audience, and Brian was petrified at the prospect of speaking to such a huge crowd. In the weeks leading up to the meeting, Brian practiced his talk relentlessly. I gave him feedback on every slide and every transition between slides. I also gave him technical tips; for example, the hand with which he held the laser pointer was prone to shaking when he was nervous, so I coached him on how to steady his pointer hand by grabbing himself around the wrist with his other hand.

On the day of the big talk, Brian seemed like he was on the verge of a panic attack. I spent a full hour before the plenary session getting him pumped up and trying to fill him with positive energy. Nonetheless, when Brian took the stage, he was shaking visibly. As the talk progressed, he began sweating profusely, with dark wet spots appearing across several areas of his shirt. He completely forgot the wrist-steadying trick I taught him, and his laser pointer was going everywhere; audience members along the edges were taking evasive action to avoid getting blinded. It was painful to watch, but Brian hung tough and made it all the way through to the end.

When Brian finished his talk, he walked off the stage and sat down next to me in the front row. He was drenched, looking like a soldier who had just come off the battlefield. I shook his hand, which was wet and clammy.

"How was it?" Brian asked.

I wanted to be encouraging, but I also didn't want to lie to him. I put my arm around him and leaned in.

"Brian," I said, "That was the best talk you could have given."

Brian smiled. This line would become a running joke between us for years to come.

I worked hard to promote Brian and the other members of my lab, and at the same time I also pushed them hard. Our discovery of the gene sequence for the beta-2 receptor, and the realization it could serve as a key to decode the sequences of other receptors, gave us a competitive advantage over other labs. However, this advantage would not last. Many other labs were jumping into the fray and using our published sequences to hunt for receptor genes, so we had to strike while the iron was hot during this brief window while we had a slight jump on the field. I pushed myself hard during this period, working late into the night and rising early to begin again. The long hours put a strain on my marriage, as I simply wasn't spending as much time with Arna and the family as I had in earlier years. In addition to burning the midnight oil myself, I exhorted my trainees to give their all. The level of intensity in the lab on a daily basis was extraordinary.

When things didn't go well in the lab, I often needed to blow off some steam. Specifically, I needed a scapegoat, and my go-to scapegoat became Henrik Dohlman, a graduate student with a sunny disposition. Even if Henrik had nothing to do with whatever problem had occurred—*especially* if Henrik had nothing to do with it—as a running lab joke I would order him to my office and fire him on the spot with great ceremony.

"Hen-Dog, you're fired!" I would yell loud enough for everyone to hear, using my preferred nickname for Henrik.

"Okay, boss!" he would chirp, then return to his lab bench and make a show of starting to pack his belongings. After a minute, I would call him back to my office again.

"Hen-Dog, you're rehired," I would say. "But don't let it happen again." I must've fired Henrik thirty or forty times during his graduate school career, and he always cheerfully went along with the joke. I don't know why, but somehow I found this repeated firing of Henrik to be oddly therapeutic. Henrik would go on to have a very successful research career, including serving as the chair of Pharmacology at the University of North Carolina, so he was apparently unharmed by the repeated firings he experienced in graduate school.

I was intense about the ongoing projects during this period and equally intense about the writing of papers. I felt like we were racing month after month to publish reports about all the new receptors and novel mechanisms of regulation we were discovering, so we needed to push the papers out rapidly or risk getting scooped by competitors. While writing the manuscript describing our identification of the beta-1 receptor, my postdoc Tom Frielle had a case of writer's block and was slow in getting me a first draft. During one of our weekly meetings that summer, he asked me with great trepidation if he could take a week off because he was planning to take his wife to the beach.

"Which beach?" I asked.

"Emerald Isle," he answered. "We're planning to share a cottage with Brian and Tong Sun and their kids."

"Sounds fun," I said. "Tell you what—you can go as long as you can get me a draft of the beta-1 manuscript before you leave."

Tom accepted this condition and began working hard to finish the draft of the manuscript before he left town that Saturday. During the week, I schmoozed with Tom and Brian a bit more and learned exactly where they were staying in Emerald Isle (a beach on the North Carolina coast) and also what realty company they were using for their rental. What I *didn't* tell them was that I was also going to Emerald Isle that week, taking my family on a beach vacation that we had booked many months earlier. Serendipitously, I was also leaving town on Saturday and happened to be using the same realty company as Tom and Brian.

On Friday, Tom gave me a draft of the beta-1 receptor manuscript. On Saturday, I drove my family to the Carolina coast. While I was picking up the keys to my rental cottage, I made an inquiry with the attendant.

"Hey, some very good friends of mine are staying here this weekend. Their names are Frielle and Kobilka. Could you please let me know if they've checked in? I'd like to stop by to say hello."

"Yes, they checked in an hour ago," said the attendant. "Cottage 14, right down on the beach." I thanked the attendant and drove my family to our cottage. After unpacking, I told Arna and the kids that I had a brief errand to run, then drove over to Cottage 14.

I wheeled into the driveway honking my horn furiously. As I approached the house, Brian, Tom, and their wives stepped out onto the deck to see what the commotion was about. I jumped out of the vehicle, brandishing the manuscript that Tom had given me the day before. I hadn't actually worked on the manuscript yet, but they didn't know that as I stormed toward the house.

"Guys, how's it going? I just drove down here to give you the latest draft of the manuscript. I gotta get back to Durham, though, so I can't stay long."

The four of them were slack-jawed. The expression on Tom's face was especially priceless, a mixture of horror and disbelief. He was probably thinking: did this psychopath really just drive three hours to give me the next draft of a manuscript that I just gave him yesterday? Naturally, I let everyone in on the joke after a few seconds and told them I happened to be staying with my family in a cottage over the ridge. I promised not to bother them again during the week and wished them a relaxing vacation.

◆

In parallel with my lab's efforts to identify the gene sequences for the adrenergic receptors and other types of receptors, we were also striving to understand the nature of receptor desensitization. The term "desensitization" refers to a loss of sensitivity to stimulation by hormones such as adrenaline. I was interested in desensitization from my earliest days in research, as this phenomenon is related to one of the most fundamental principles in all of physiology: the principle of homeostasis. If you perturb a cell, by overstimulating with adrenaline or anything else, that cell is going to do everything it can to get back to the condition it was in before you perturbed it. Desensitization of receptor signaling is a central way that all cells maintain homeostasis.

Our earliest studies on desensitization revealed that when cells were overstimulated with adrenaline or other beta receptor activators, there was an apparent small increase in beta receptor size as determined by one particular technique. These observations mystified us, and in the early 1980s I showed these findings during a Howard Hughes workshop in Coconut Grove, Florida. In the audience that day was a fellow Hughes investigator named Ed Krebs, who years later would win the

Nobel Prize for the discovery of protein phosphorylation (i.e., the addition of phosphate groups to proteins as a major mechanism of cellular regulation). Ed was normally a very low-key fellow, but when he saw my data he suddenly became highly animated. I had never seen the guy so excited; he literally jumped out of his seat and spoke up.

"Bob, I'll tell you *exactly* what's causing that size change," he said breathlessly. "Your receptor is being phosphorylated!" Ed went on to say that he knew from his own lab's work that when phosphate groups were added to a protein, there was often a small but detectable increase in apparent size, similar to the apparent increase in size we saw in the beta-2 receptor following stimulation. At the time, nobody had ever examined phosphorylation of receptors, so the idea seemed radical. However, Krebs seemed sure of himself, so I leapt into action.

Immediately after the session, I called Jeff Stadel, the postdoc who was spearheading my lab's work on desensitization. I told him that Ed Krebs was certain our receptor was being phosphorylated in a manner that might correlate with desensitization, and I proposed that we obtain some radiolabeled phosphate to check this idea. To make a long story short: Jeff and others in my lab checked it out and found that the beta receptor was indeed phosphorylated. Subsequently, with this project being carried forward over the years by Ponnal Nambi, Berta Strulovici, David Sibley, Michel Bouvier, and others, we found evidence that this phosphorylation was not only correlated with desensitization, but was actually part of the mechanism that caused it.[5]

Given the importance of this receptor phosphorylation, the next pressing task was to figure out exactly how phosphates were getting added to the beta receptor. Phosphates don't magically attach to things inside a cell; they must be actively attached by an enzyme called a "kinase." In the mid-1980s, Jeff Benovic, a graduate student in my lab, took an interest in trying to purify the kinase that was so powerfully regulating the beta receptor. In Jeff's first year in my lab, he had an abstract accepted to present a poster at a big national meeting, and then received a letter stating that because his abstract might be of public interest, he needed to make himself available at the meeting to talk to reporters. I jokingly bestowed the nickname "Scoop" on Jeff because he was such a media darling. Over the course of the next week, though, one by one every member of my lab who had submitted an abstract to this meeting eventually received the same letter. Later, we learned that every single poster presenter at the meeting had received exactly the same letter as Scoop, but somehow the nickname still stuck.

Over a period of several years, Scoop painstakingly figured out how to purify the kinase that was attaching phosphates to the beta receptor to induce desensitization.[6] We initially named this enzyme the beta-adrenergic receptor kinase (BARK for short). This breakthrough led to the realization that receptors for many (if not all) hormones become phosphorylated as a key step in their process of desensitization, further demonstrating the power of the beta receptor gene sequence as a Rosetta Stone. Indeed, our appreciation of the similarity between the beta receptor and rhodopsin led rapidly to another key insight. In 1987, just a year after our discovery of the similarity of the beta receptor and rhodopsin, a protein called "arrestin" was shown to be important for desensitization of rhodopsin. However, arrestin was only found in the retina, so we speculated that there must be similar proteins that played analogous roles for other receptors outside the eye. We ultimately identified two so-called "beta-arrestins," and the gene sequences for these nonvisual arrestins were worked out by Martin Lohse, Håvard Attramadal, Jeff Benovic, and others in the lab.[7] We discovered that the beta-arrestins bound to the receptors after phosphorylation, thereby preventing receptor stimulation of G proteins, with the result being desensitization.

◆

Einstein had his *annus mirabilis* ("miraculous year") in 1905, when he published four distinct papers—on Brownian motion, special relativity, mass-energy equivalence, and the photoelectric effect—and each paper was a breakthrough worthy of a Nobel Prize. I don't pretend to be in the same league as Einstein, but when I look back over my career it's clear that my *annus mirabilis* was 1986–87. In a little over a year, we cloned the beta-2 receptor gene, discovered its architectural similarity to the visual signaling molecule rhodopsin, and also discovered the kinase that phosphorylates the beta-2 receptor and the beta-arrestins that bound the receptor to lead to its desensitization. These interconnected discoveries, culminating more than fifteen years of work, represented the first glimpse of what eventually would be known as the superfamily of G protein–coupled receptors, the largest gene family in the human genome, a constellation of related receptors operating with conserved principles. During that miraculous year of 1986–87, and for several years afterward, I was riding a wave of professional success that was intoxicating and all-consuming. I pushed myself hard and also pushed the members of my lab to keep striving for new heights. Soaring peaks are often followed by deep valleys, however, and it turned out that I was about to descend into one of the darkest valleys of my life.

FIFTEEN

How to Fix a Broken Heart

I came home from work one night in 1989 and Arna said, *"We need to talk."* Those four words are usually a harbinger of a difficult conversation. Indeed, with very little preamble, Arna told me that she wanted to separate. The marriage had been rocky for several years, although she found it difficult to articulate exactly what was wrong. Given the issues we'd been having, I should not have been all that surprised, but in the moment, it seemed to come out of the blue, and I was devastated.

For as long as I could remember, my life had revolved around two centers, my family and my work. I was passionate about my career, first as a physician and then as a scientist, and there's no doubt that the long hours I spent pursuing this passion cut into time spent with my family. Arna never stated this directly, but in retrospect I assumed this must have been the core issue. And so at midlife, I suddenly found myself confronted with the classic "midlife crisis." When it happens to someone else, it's a cliché, but when it happens to you, it's a tragedy. I felt like a failure. For months after that conversation, I was a wreck.

Arna and I separated, and then ultimately divorced a year later. Despite the intensity of the emotions involved, the divorce was as amicable as divorces can be. Arna and I had been high school sweethearts, but during the separation it became clear that we now wanted different things and were moving in different directions. Our kids were all out of the house except for Josh, who was twelve at that time. We came to an agreement about how Josh's time would be shared, and the other kids were all understanding about the split.

During this difficult period, I leaned heavily on my friends, especially Ralph Snyderman. We ran together every day, and he was like my therapist. Ralph's lab had been just down the hall from mine for many years—in an earlier chapter, I described how Ralph and I enjoyed trading "war stories" about our time at the NIH as Yellow Berets. Ralph had left Duke for several years to become a vice president for Research at Genentech, but then returned to Duke in 1989 as both the dean of the School of Medicine and chancellor for Health Affairs. Upon his return to Duke, he also resumed his role as my main running partner. Ralph listened patiently to me mile after mile as I sorted out my feelings. During difficult times like going through a divorce, there's nothing more important than having close friends to act as sounding boards. Talking to Ralph every day helped keep me sane.

◆

The years following the divorce marked the beginning of my cardiac troubles. Every morning it was the same: I experienced chest tightness for the first mile of the run, but then it would go away as the run progressed. During the cooldown period, the tightness would return. I kept telling myself that this couldn't be angina, because it went away during the run. As a cardiologist, though, I should've recognized this was actually a classic pattern of exercise-induced angina. It turned out that my training in cardiology was no match for my astonishing powers of self-delusion.

I experienced angina on my runs for months, and my main response was to increase the intensity of my workouts. In hindsight, this was crazy, but somehow I thought I could just push through it. It was as if I was literally trying to run away from my family history of heart troubles. At fifty, I was now the same age my father had been when he had his first heart attack, a fact that was very much on my mind. When I finally admitted to Ralph in the spring of 1994 that I was experiencing chest tightness during our runs together, he insisted that I had to get it checked, especially given my horrific family history.

I made an appointment to see our colleague Jim Morris. Jim recommended a radionuclide test, which involves running on a treadmill and getting injected with a dye to image the heart during exercise. During the test, an electrocardiogram (EKG) is also performed. When I came off the treadmill, I took a quick look at my own EKG and saw evidence that my heart was experiencing significant ischemia, meaning that parts of the cardiac muscle were not getting enough oxygen. After the test, I asked Jim what he thought, but he hemmed and hawed and declined to answer, saying he needed to look over all the results. The next morning, he called me into his office and said things didn't look good. He recommended a cardiac catheterization to get a better view of what was going on.

I felt profoundly depressed after speaking with Jim. I had been a hypochondriac my whole life, and it had served me well: I was always fearing that something terrible was wrong with me, but then I'd get it checked out and find it was actually nothing. Thus, despite having angina for months, despite my own reading of the EKG, I had still been hoping against hope that Jim was going to say, *"Hey, Bob, I looked things over and it's not that bad. You've been worrying for no reason."* Instead, he'd said, *"This doesn't look good."* I happened to be hosting a visit that day from Rick Cerione, my former postdoc who was now a faculty member at Cornell. When I introduced Rick at his seminar, I tried to put up a cheerful front, but my colleagues (including Rick) could tell that something was wrong. I was deeply, deeply worried about what the cardiac catheterization procedure might reveal.

The cath procedure was performed by my friend Dave Kong. As described at the beginning of Chapter 1, the last thing I saw as the anesthesia kicked in was my coronary arteries lighting up due to calcium deposits, which often accompany severe atherosclerosis. After I uttered *"Oh, shit"* and conked out, I woke up in the recovery room and then waited for what seemed like forever. I was on pins and needles waiting for Jim Morris to walk into the room and tell me what was going on. An eternity passed, and finally Jim did come in, but he was not alone: he was accompanied by five additional colleagues, including Dave Kong and the entire leadership of the cardiology division. I was thinking, *"What the hell is going on?"* It felt like an intervention.

"Bob, you have complex coronary artery disease," Jim said. "It's two-vessel disease—both the left and right vessels have multiple significant lesions. Also, one of the diagonal branches off your left anterior descending coronary artery is 100 percent occluded. Stenting is not feasible. You're going to need bypass surgery."

My thoughts were racing and I had a hundred technical questions. This was the reason why they had brought the whole team into the room—they figured I might try to argue with Jim and question his interpretation. However, if all of these heavy hitters stood shoulder to shoulder recommending the same treatment plan, it would be harder for me to resist. Eventually, after an extended discussion, I capitulated. I was headed for quadruple bypass surgery.[1]

For scheduling reasons, the surgery would be performed in two weeks. These two weeks I felt the most anxious I ever have in my entire life. A coronary bypass is an intense procedure, and a lot of things can go wrong.

To help deal with my anxiety, I rigorously prepared for the surgery. For example, I spoke with my colleague David Sabiston, who at that time was the chair of the Surgery Department and one of the most legendary heart surgeons in the world. I asked David: if *he* were having a bypass at Duke, who would he want to do it? David recommended Peter Van Trigt, a cardiac surgeon I didn't know but who apparently was the most skilled coronary bypass specialist on the Duke campus. I requested that Van Trigt perform my surgery, and when I met with him found that he had a very dry, reserved personality. I shared my thoughts about him with Jim Morris, who smiled.

"Well, Bob, let's just say we didn't hire him for his personality. We hired this guy for his hands!"

During the two-week wait, I also got in touch with Jerry Reves, the chair of Anesthesiology at Duke. Jerry was a renowned cardiac anesthesiologist and very good friend of mine, so I asked if he could personally handle my anesthesia. He said that he had plans to be on vacation with his wife that week on an island off the South Carolina coast, but for me he would fly back to Duke for a couple of days in the middle of his vacation to handle the anesthesia and make sure that everything went well in the post-op period. Now that's friendship! I slept better in the days leading up to the procedure knowing that Jerry would be in the operating room with me.

◆

The interminable two-week wait before the bypass surgery was a time of deep personal reflection for me. The preceding several years of my life had been very eventful. Professionally, I was on top of the world, publishing important papers, winning awards, and traveling the globe to give invited lectures. Personally, though, it had been a turbulent period.

After my divorce from Arna, I had gone through a period of intense soul searching. For the first time in my life, I began keeping a journal. The opening entry of this journal read: *"My entire adult life has been colored by two deeply-held beliefs: one, that I would die young, and two, that I would accomplish something of real significance."* After my diagnosis of coronary artery disease in 1994, this journal entry seemed prescient. I wondered if my work as a researcher to that point would be remembered in the eyes of history as a contribution of real significance, and also wondered how many more years (if any) I would be able to keep adding to that body of work.

Fortunately, I did not have to face the bypass surgery completely alone. In the preceding years, my running group with Ralph Snyderman and others had been joined on occasion by Lynn Tilley, who many years earlier had worked with me as an administrative assistant at Duke. She had left Duke in 1984, completed a degree in psychology at the University of North Carolina, and then pursued her career. When she joined the running group, we developed a strong friendship. We had always gotten along well when we had a strictly professional relationship years before, but during our many hours together running on the roads we bonded in a new way. Lynn had a remarkably empathetic way of listening as I spoke of my concerns and tribulations. Also, as a neurotic New York Jew, I found her easygoing Southern ways refreshing. Following my divorce, this friendship with Lynn eventually deepened into romance, and a couple of years later, we were married.

After my heart disease diagnosis, Lynn was a rock for me. She was with me in the recovery room when that large group of my colleagues had given me the bad news. She was by my side during all the preparations for the surgery. As a physician myself, I was acutely aware that major surgeries like bypasses can be just as tough on spouses as on the patients themselves. I felt fortunate to have Lynn in the foxhole with me as I prepared for what was to come.

On the day of my bypass surgery, I was awakened in my hospital bed at 5:30 A.M. and shaved by a nurse from head to foot. I was wheeled into the operating room where my friend Jerry was waiting to administer the anesthesia. We made small talk about his vacation, and then the anesthesia kicked in and the next thing I knew I was waking up in the recovery room. I was told that the surgery went well, although later I would learn a detail that scared the hell out of me. During a coronary bypass, it is necessary to arrest the cardiac muscle so that the surgeon doesn't have to operate on a beating, squirming heart. While the heart is stopped, the patient is kept alive using a heart-lung machine (technically known as a cardiopulmonary bypass machine). Then, when the procedure is finished, the heart is restarted by electric shock. In my case, the heart did not restart on the first shock, and in fact didn't resume beating until the *fourth* electric shock. I was unnerved when I learned this information.[2] What if my heart had never restarted? It was as if I had died on the operating table and then been resurrected.

Waking up after the surgery was a surreal experience. I had more lines in my body than I thought possible: two different IV lines, pacing wires in my heart, a tube down my throat, four chest tubes, a catheter in my bladder, and for good measure my chest was fully covered with electrodes. I was doped up on drugs and lights were flashing everywhere. It was like being trapped in a crazy dream.

Shortly after I awoke, I was visited by Ralph Snyderman. Normally visitors would not be allowed at this time, but Ralph was in charge of the whole medical center, so nobody could stop him.

"Bob, is there anything I can do for you?" Ralph asked. I couldn't speak, because I was intubated, so one of the nurses handed me a piece of paper, on which I wrote, *"Get the damn tube out!"* I wrote these words vertically rather than horizontally, because I was spaced out from the drugs. Ralph laughed and said he would see what he could do, and a short time later I was able to breathe well enough to have the tube removed. I was then moved to the intensive care unit (ICU).

They say doctors make the worst patients, and I was definitely a bad patient. Physicians are used to being in control and thus find it hard to let someone else call the shots. Worse, we seek multiple opinions from our colleagues, who *never* agree on the best plan. Indeed, the nurses in the ICU were driven crazy by my constant stream of visitors, as one after another of my cardiology colleagues made their way to see me and offered unsolicited commentary on how my recovery plan was being handled. Finally, the head nurse said, *"If you get one more visitor, I don't care who it is, I'm going to grab them by the scruff of the neck and throw them out of here."* Right at that moment, Ralph Snyderman walked through the door again, which would've made me laugh except that my chest hurt too much. The nurse did not carry out her threat to grab the dean of the medical school by the scruff of his neck, and he was allowed to stay.

Despite the drugs I was being given, my chest still hurt like hell. At the start of the bypass surgery, my chest had been cut completely open (called a "sternotomy") and then put back together when the bypass was done. These days, so-called "keyhole" bypasses can be performed using much less invasive procedures that do not involve cutting open the sternum, but such techniques had not yet been developed in 1994. Thus, I needed heavy doses of painkillers and knew I was destined for a long road to recovery.

After a week, I was finally able to leave the hospital. Lynn took me home, helped me into our bed, and turned on the television. I was still taking high doses of opiates, Xanax, and several other drugs, so I was heavily medicated and trying hard to process what I was seeing on TV. I was watching a white SUV driving along a deserted freeway, with dozens of police cars following behind. This scene seemed to go on for a very long time with few plot developments, so finally I turned to Lynn in a state of confusion.

"What movie is this?" I asked.

"This is not a movie," she answered. "This is O. J. Simpson being chased by the police."

"WHAT?" I exclaimed. "Did I miss something while I was in the hospital?" Lynn then patiently filled me in on recent news, including the Simpson murder case.

In my first few weeks back home, I developed significant anxiety and depression, which is not uncommon in patients following major operations such as open-heart surgeries. I became very dependent on Lynn and felt anxious whenever she left the room. My brain wasn't working well, so even if she left for just a minute I would become fearful that she wasn't returning and start dreading that I might drop dead at any moment. Lynn was patient with me and gave me a whistle that I could blow if I was having any problems when she was out of the room. Somehow, having the whistle nearby made me feel better.

Slowly but surely, with Lynn's untiring help, I was able to get over the anxiety and depression, but my cognitive abilities remained fuzzy. After long surgeries like bypasses, some patients report mental fogginess that persists for weeks or months, sometimes indefinitely. I became concerned that I might be one of those patients who had lost a bit of high-end cognitive ability that would not be regained. Moreover, I recalled that when my father began having his heart troubles, at the very same age I was now, he slowed down both physically and mentally, as if his malfunctioning heart was sucking the life force out of him. I was fearful that this might be happening to me as well, which meant that the torpor and fuzziness I was experiencing might persist as a permanent condition.

Despite my lingering cognitive slowness, I began having some of my students and postdoctoral fellows visit the house to discuss their research projects with me. I was going through data withdrawal and feeling anxious to know what had been going on in the lab in my absence. Moreover, I felt badly about abandoning all the young scientists in my lab, which at that time had more than twenty people. Thus, even though I still wasn't 100 percent and couldn't physically make it into the lab, I invited the lab members to my house to talk about their latest findings.

After one such visit, Lynn walked the visitors out of the house and then came back into the kitchen to find me crying.

"Bob, what's wrong?" she asked with deep concern.

"Nothing is wrong," I said as tears rolled down my cheeks. "Nothing at all. I just realized that my brain is working again."

I had felt mentally sharp during the session with my students and had been able to follow every word they had said. I also had been able to offer significant insights into their projects, even recalling specific scientific papers that the students should read to help understand their data. It was the first time since the surgery that my brain felt like it was returning to normal, and I was overwhelmed with joy. I just sat there in the kitchen, sobbing uncontrollably with relief. My brain was back, and I was ready to return to action.

SIXTEEN

Against the Odds

After I fully recovered from my bypass surgery, I became more committed than ever to my daily runs. Over the course of many months, I ramped my mileage back up to pre-surgery levels. Some of my colleagues and acquaintances were amused by my renewed passion for running. In my early days back at work after the bypass surgery, one particularly insensitive colleague had teased me about my dedication to my exercise regimen.

"Hey, Bob, I guess all that running didn't do you any good," my colleague said. "You still needed a quadruple bypass!"

My response to such naïve comments was to argue that, in fact, running had saved my life. The cath exam prior to my bypass had revealed that several branches of my coronary arteries were severely narrowed, and one major branch was *completely* occluded. Normally, such a total blockage would cause a heart attack. However, the cath also revealed that I had robust collateral circulation, which was shunting blood around the blocked area. My collateral circulation in these regions was almost certainly the result of my exercise regimen: when an area of the heart muscle is not getting enough oxygen, as can happen in a heart with narrowed arteries during strenuous workouts, the heart responds by building extra blood vessels to provide additional blood flow. In my case, these extra vessels prevented a heart attack.

The increased intensity of my exercise regimen following my quadruple bypass surgery was the exact opposite of the approach my father had taken after his heart attacks. His doctors had ordered him to cease all strenuous physical activity in order to protect his heart. Subsequent research has proven that regular exercise strongly promotes cardiac health. In fact, exercise significantly reduces the risk of many age-related diseases, including coronary artery disease, hypertension, diabetes, dementia and several types of cancer. If there were a pill that could confer the health benefits of exercise, every single person on the planet would take this pill. In the absence of such a pill, however, I ramped up my running.

My workout routine was strengthened by the fact that I had terrific training partners. I'm a very social person, so having training partners with whom to schmooze during workouts has always made the experience infinitely more enjoyable for me. When I first began running during my residency at Columbia and service at the NIH, I honestly didn't enjoy it very much. I only developed a true passion for running during my senior residency and cardiology fellowship at Mass General, when I began meeting up with a simpatico group of friends for daily morning runs along the Charles River in Boston. After I moved to Duke, I continued to enjoy running in a group, with my most consistent training partner both before and after my bypass surgery being Ralph Snyderman. The only reasons Ralph and I ever canceled runs were due to lightning or ice; otherwise, we ran. We ran as a pair, we ran in large groups, and we even ran together on the coldest day in the history of North Carolina (-9 degrees Fahrenheit), a feat that required both of us to be fully clad in elaborate ski gear, which I had to borrow from Ralph since I didn't ski. Ralph once calculated that if you added up all of our shared miles, we ran more than twice around the globe together.

My longest run ever with Ralph was a twenty-mile sojourn with our friend Norm Silverman. At the start of this run, we noticed we were being stalked by a mangy wild dog. The dog's intentions were uncertain; we wondered if perhaps he was planning to track us until we dropped and then feast on our carcasses. We tried to scare him off by shouting, gesticulating wildly, and throwing sticks, all to no avail. As the run progressed, we kept a wary eye on our canine companion, even as the conversation drifted to other topics.

We schmoozed about our recent training sessions with the legendary Stu Mittleman. Stu was one of the greatest ultramarathoners of all time, having set numerous world records in races between 100 and 1,000 miles in distance. He had been living and training in the Raleigh-Durham area, and Ralph and I somehow became part of Stu's expansive cohort of training partners. Stu needed a lot of partners because he ran thirty or forty miles *per day*. No single person could keep up with him the entire time, so he would rotate through groups of running buddies who would accompany him for ten- or fifteen-mile stretches. The previous week, when Ralph and I had finished a run with Stu, he hadn't even stopped to say goodbye: he'd just kept on running as the next wave of training partners tagged in.

As Ralph, Norm, and I traded stories, we completed our twenty-mile run and slowed to a stop. We were totally exhausted. The dog was still with us, having followed us the entire time. It had become clear that he was friendly, and now he stood in front of us panting as a smile creased his face. He was looking at us like, *"You guys aren't done already, are you? I'm just getting warmed up."* He then loped off down the trail in search of his next group of runners. He seemed content and happy being free.

"That dog reminds me of Stu Mittleman," I said, as Ralph and Norm laughed in agreement.

Ralph and I were best friends, but also very competitive. When we were apart due to travel, I would still keep up my daily training runs because I wanted to get in better shape than Ralph. He and I ran many road races together, with Ralph always winning, so I became increasingly desperate to beat Ralph just once. After my bypass surgery, I worked as hard as I could to get back in racing shape, biding my time for an opportunity to take Ralph down. In a 10 km race around the Duke campus one morning, I finally had my chance. Just past the 5 km mark, I was surprised to suddenly see Ralph by the side of the road on his hands and knees. As I approached, I called out to him.

"Ralph, what's wrong?"

"I lost my key!" he shouted as he groped the pavement.

Perhaps I should have stopped to help my friend in his moment of need. However, I saw an opportunity to finally beat Ralph in a race, so I put the pedal to the metal and blasted past him. With a half-mile to go, I was still ahead of him and feeling great. Suddenly, from out of nowhere, Ralph came powering past and beat me by a few seconds. After the race, I felt guilty for abandoning Ralph by the side of the road—and he still beat me!—but he said he understood and in fact would do the same thing if the circumstances were reversed. I continued training hard with the goal of beating Ralph, even though I knew that such a golden opportunity would probably never come around again.

I have always loved stories of people striving against the odds. As a kid, I read biographies of Winston Churchill and Abraham Lincoln, feeling moved by their resolute leadership at moments when everything seemed lost. Similarly, I love stories about mountain climbers who persevere to reach their peaks despite the loss of equipment, fingers, and fellow climbers. I love unstoppable runners like Stu Mittleman (and the Mittleman-esque feral dog) because they exemplify toughness, hanging in there for as long as they can and never giving up. After my bypass surgery, I began to see myself as an underdog who was bucking the odds and battling hard to hang in there. I had been dealt an unfortunate hand in terms of cardiovascular risk factors inherited from my parents, but I was determined to beat the odds and be a survivor.

◆

Exercise was not the only approach I took in trying to defuse the time bomb in my chest. During my medicine sub-internship at Goldwater Memorial Hospital in 1965, I gave blood for a study on lipids and learned that my total blood cholesterol level was 260. At the time, this was not particularly troubling to me, as a clear link between blood levels of cholesterol and atherosclerotic vascular disease had not yet been established. In the early 1980s, a blood sample was drawn during a routine annual physical and I was again told that my cholesterol was over 250. By that time, there had been multiple studies suggesting that cholesterol levels higher than 200 were linked to cardiovascular disease, so my Duke colleagues raised alarm bells over my high cholesterol readings. It seemed probable that my high cholesterol levels were due partly to genetics, which were likely a major contributor to my family history of heart attacks and other cardiac disease. However, diet was also certainly a factor, as I ate a standard American diet of the era, including plenty of McDonald's and other fast food offerings with my young children.

Following my quadruple bypass surgery, I developed a totally different mindset about my diet. I was heavily influenced by the writings of the cardiologist Dean Ornish on the benefits of reducing fat intake. Ornish wrote a best-selling book called *Dr. Dean Ornish's Program for Reversing Heart Disease*, which recommended a stringent low-fat diet as a means of combating coronary artery disease and atherosclerosis. However, I was also influenced by other studies of this era demonstrating that not all fats were created equal: saturated fats can raise "bad" LDL cholesterol levels, but mono- and polyunsaturated fats can actually help to reduce LDL cholesterol values. Thus, I began an Ornish-style diet that evolved over time into an almost-vegan diet featuring lots of vegetables, fruits, whole grains, beans, nuts, and olive oil. This transition was not difficult since Lynn was a vegetarian, so by association I also became vegetarian, finding like most vegetarians that I didn't miss meat at all. The eating plan that Lynn and I evolved over time was very low in saturated fats, although not especially low in overall fats.

Once this dietary regimen was in place, I never wavered from it. I was zealously observant even when eating out at professional events, which sometimes prompted colleagues to comment on my strict adherence to my diet.

"Bob, are you sure don't want to try the dessert? It's amazing. You don't know what you're missing!"

In truth, I had no problem adhering to my new diet because I didn't think of myself as "on a diet." I grew up in a kosher home. Even when my family ate out, we observed kashrut, the set of dietary laws dealing with foods that Jews are permitted to eat and how those foods must be prepared. In observing kashrut, you either observed the dietary laws or you didn't; there was no in-between. You didn't eat a pork chop or ham sandwich every once in a while just because it was a special occasion. "Diets" are things you cheat on and eventually go off. When I made the commitment to eat healthier after my bypass surgery, I viewed myself as similar to an orthodox Jew following kashrut: I wasn't on a diet, I just ate a different way than most people.

Given my inherited predisposition to high cholesterol, my healthy diet could only reduce my bad cholesterol levels so far. To reduce levels further, I took advantage of several recently developed drugs. I had already been taking lovastatin (Mevacor) since its approval by the FDA in 1987. This drug was the first "statin" to be approved for medical use, and it lowers cholesterol levels by inhibiting the activity of HMG-CoA reductase, the rate-limiting enzyme required for the synthesis of cholesterol. Later, I would begin taking even more powerful statins, such as rosuvastatin (Crestor), as well as an additional drug, ezetimibe, which blocks uptake of cholesterol in the small intestine. I started keeping obsessive track of my cholesterol values and found it very satisfying to watch my cholesterol numbers descend to subterranean levels. This made me feel empowered, as if I were actively combating cardiovascular disease in real time in a manner that could be measured. Moreover, since I was directing a research laboratory but no longer personally doing experiments at the bench during this time, I enjoyed tracking my cholesterol numbers because it provided the only data I was capable of generating myself.

I kept elaborate spreadsheets of all my cholesterol values. Whenever I made changes to my exercise regimen, diet, or medication, I would meticulously look for concomitant changes in my cholesterol numbers. The goal of this self-experimentation was to help me drive my LDL cholesterol levels as low as possible. One day, a cardiology fellow in my lab asked if he could use my remarkably complete personal data set for a teaching conference on hypercholesterolemia that he had to present to a group of Duke cardiology fellows the following week. He assured me that he wouldn't reveal who the patient in question was.

"Sure, you can use my data," I told him. "On the condition that I get to attend the session as a faculty discussant."

At the conference, the cardiology fellow from my lab played up how obsessive this patient must be to collect so much detailed data. The other fellows agreed and made numerous snide and sarcastic comments about this obviously neurotic patient. I laughed along with the group and we had a very informative, educational, and enjoyable conference. When it was over, the fellows asked me as a faculty member if I had any final comments to complete the discussion. I made a few technical comments about the nuances of medical treatments for high cholesterol and then made a brief closing statement.

"By the way, the patient is me."

The room fell silent, save for a few nervous laughs. I have to confess that I enjoyed the discomfiture all the fellows experienced upon hearing this revelation. Perhaps in the future they would think twice before cracking jokes about patients during clinical conferences.

In addition to cholesterol-lowering drugs, I also took medications to control another cardiovascular risk factor that I inherited from my parents: high blood pressure. I took both enalapril, an inhibitor of angiotensin-converting enzyme (ACE), and atenolol, a beta blocker. It was admittedly somewhat ironic that I began blocking my beta-adrenergic receptors on a daily basis to render them less sensitive to my body's output of adrenaline, given that my signature research discovery was showing how adrenaline acts through beta receptors. However, my goal was to defy genetics and stay alive as long as possible, and beta blockers were helping me to achieve this goal.

It's worth noting that all of the drugs I was taking to lower my cholesterol and blood pressure were developed in part based on research funded by the National Institutes of Health. The development of these and many other life-saving drugs is a wonderful example of our tax dollars being well spent. Statins, beta blockers, ACE inhibitors, and cholesterol-uptake inhibitors collectively save millions of lives around the world each year. Not a single one of these drugs was around in the 1950s when my father was beginning to have his heart problems. If these drugs had been around at that time, there's a good chance my dad could have lived decades longer.

I saw myself as living proof that genetics is not destiny. Through a combination of exercise, diet, and drugs, I was determined to overcome the multiple cardiovascular risk factors I inherited from my parents. I resolved to try as hard as I could to beat the odds and live as long and robust a life as possible. I had a lot to live for: I wanted to meet my grandchildren, enjoy more years with Lynn, and have more time to pursue the exciting research stories being developed in my lab. I was fired up about turning the page to the forthcoming chapters of my life. I couldn't have known it at the time, but many of the wildest years of my life were still to come.

SEVENTEEN

"Well, It's Not the Nobel Prize . . ."

I n the early morning darkness, the phone in my bedroom was ringing. The date was October 10, 1994. I was still in bed and started cursing, wondering who could be calling me at this ungodly hour. After fumbling around for a few seconds, I answered the phone with a half-mumbled *"Hello?"*

"Is this Dr. Lefkowitz?" asked a male voice.

"Yes."

"Dr. Lefkowitz, I would appreciate your comment on this morning's Nobel Prize announcement."

I paused a few seconds to let this sink in. Then I asked the obvious question.

"Did I win?"

There was a long pause on the other end. Finally, the voice spoke again.

"No," said the voice. "Sorry, but . . . uh . . . no. This morning's Nobel Prize in Physiology or Medicine was just announced for Alfred Gilman and Martin Rodbell for the discovery of G proteins. I'm a reporter with the Associated Press. Given your expertise in this area, I was hoping you could offer me some commentary about these scientists and their work."

I have to confess: I was a bit crestfallen to hear this news, but tried to hide that fact from the reporter as I provided him with some quotes about why G proteins are important. Later in the day, I dished out similar quotes to other reporters who called my office. It was a chaotic day, and I strove to maintain a placid demeanor even though inside I was churning with disappointment.

Like many people who are nominated for Nobel Prizes, I had heard rumors that my name was under consideration but tried to act like the whole Nobel thing didn't matter. I'm not a good actor, though, so I probably didn't fool many people. I was also well aware that each Nobel can be given to a maximum of three people, per an ironclad statute of the Nobel Foundation. Thus, for the Nobel Prize shared by Gilman and Rodbell, there was an extra slot available. In my mind, it was logical that I could've shared this Prize: G proteins and their receptors go together like hand and glove. By 1994, my lab had purified the first hormone receptor that acted via G proteins (the beta-2 adrenergic receptor). We had also performed the first complete reconstitution experiments, ahead of Gilman, showing that a purified system of receptor, G protein, and cyclase could mediate hormone signaling. Additionally, we had cloned the gene for the beta-2 receptor and many other receptors, discovering their structural relationship to each other (and to rhodopsin), as well as their shared mechanisms of desensitization, thereby establishing the concept of a large family of G protein–coupled receptors. Given this body of work, I felt like my lab's contributions in this area were beyond question.

I knew it was conceivable that there might be a separate Nobel Prize someday for the characterization of G protein–coupled receptors. Then again, there might not be. The Nobel committee is always so overwhelmed in considering so many important discoveries from different subfields, it's impossible for them to recognize every worthy nominee. For this reason, I felt that any chance I might have had to win a Nobel Prize had probably just gone by the boards.

Coincidentally, at my fiftieth birthday party the year before, I had been roasted by a group of lab members and alumni over whether or not I would ever win a Nobel. John Raymond, a clinical fellow in my lab, had photoshopped a fake newspaper with the headline DUKE PROFESSOR TAKES NOBEL PRIZE. The article under the headline was a story about Gilman winning the Prize and then having it stolen by me. In the article's narrative, I was eventually caught and arrested, with the final line of the article reading, *"As Lefkowitz was led away in handcuffs, he was heard mumbling something about male menopause."* This fake newspaper that John put together was quite prescient, as Gilman did indeed win the Nobel Prize the following year and it did indeed bother me. To my credit, though, my irritation over the announcement did not lead me to commit grand larceny.

Why does the Nobel Prize matter so much to scientists, and also to the public at large? These days, there are a huge number of scientific prizes, some of which come attached to much larger amounts of money than does the Nobel Prize. However, the Nobel retains a mystique that no other award can match. Part of the reason is undoubtedly historical: when the Nobel Prizes were founded in Stockholm, Sweden, in 1901, they were the first major international awards given for scientific research. No matter how much money is offered by newer prizes like the Breakthrough Prize (current prize value: $3 million), Albert Einstein will never win a Breakthrough Prize. Marie Curie will never win a Breakthrough. The fact that legends like Einstein and Curie *did* win Nobel Prizes adds luster to the Nobel that newer prizes lack. When the new Laureates are announced by the Nobel committees each October, they join an august list of former winners that is graced by some of the greatest geniuses in history.

Another reason why the Nobel Prizes stand head and shoulders above other scientific awards is because Nobel Prizes are not given just for scientific research. Nobels are also awarded for Economics, Literature, and Peace. Thus, all Nobel Prize winners in the sciences get to share the stage with illustrious writers and leaders, not to mention historical figures such as Winston Churchill, Ernest Hemingway, Martin Luther King Jr., and Mother Teresa. The fact that the Nobel Prizes are given in many different categories contributes to their wide public appeal, which cannot be matched by other prizes that are strictly given for scientific discoveries.

The renown of the Nobel Prizes is so great that even my mother, a woman who knew very little about science or scholarly activities of any kind, knew all about the Nobels. Throughout my career, whenever I won any scientific prize, my mother's response was always the same.

"Well, it's not the Nobel Prize."

I heard this refrain again and again. In 1978, when I won the prestigious Abel Award, an award given to an investigator under the age of forty who makes outstanding research contributions in biology, I remember my mother's response was, *"Well, that's nice, Bobby, but it's not the Nobel Prize."* She would subsequently repeat this phrase on many other occasions when being informed of any award I had received. For my mother, it was apparently the Nobel or bust. This was one reason why it stung a bit to not share the Nobel Prize in 1994: my mother's health was in a downward spiral at that time and I feared she wouldn't live much longer. After a lifetime of hearing that my achievements were "nice" but not at the Nobel level, it would've been very satisfying to take my mom to Stockholm to show her that I had finally made good.

My mother's health had been deteriorating for a number of years. In 1986, my mom was still living in the same rent-controlled apartment in the Bronx that I grew up in. One night, I got a call from my Aunt Pauline saying that my mother had been rushed to the hospital because she was having trouble breathing. My mother had been suffering from a number of cardiac issues and had gone into acute heart failure with pulmonary edema, which was the proximal cause of her breathing issues. When I heard the news from Aunt Pauline, I packed my stethoscope and headed to the airport to catch the first available flight to New York City.

I examined my mother myself the next day and consulted with the doctors at Albert Einstein Medical Center, where she was staying. The diagnosis was aortic stenosis, a narrowing of the aortic valve. If left untreated, she would probably be dead in a year or two. However, a surgery to replace her aortic valve might prolong her life by a decade or more. I had done my residency across town at Columbia-Presbyterian and still had many contacts there, and I knew Columbia had a great team in place performing aortic valve replacements. Thus, I arranged for my mother to be transferred to Columbia for her surgery, which would be an aortic valve replacement in addition to a triple coronary artery bypass. The aortic valve transplant that she received came from a pig, and when she woke up from her surgery she looked at me with a serious gaze and said, *"Bobby, I'm not kosher anymore."*

After getting out of the hospital, my mother's health stabilized for almost a decade but then took another downturn in 1995, a year after my own bypass surgery. I moved my mother from Florida, where she had been living with my Aunt Pauline, to a nursing home in Durham, just a mile from the Duke campus. I sensed that my mother didn't have much time left and I wanted to make sure that I could spend some extra time with her.

After my mother's move to Durham, I visited her every single day. I would religiously leave my office at Duke at 6:00 P.M. each evening and arrive at the nursing home precisely at 6:10. When I walked into my mother's room, she would look at her huge watch, which had oversized numbers because her eyes were failing, then look up at me and say, *"It's about time!"*

"Ma, I come at the same exact time every day!" I would say in exasperation. She would just shrug.

We would hang out and talk for a bit, then watch the evening news. My mother's heart, liver, and kidneys were failing, but her mind was still sharp. She did the *New York Times* crossword puzzle every day, so we would talk about that day's puzzle and also discuss the evening news, as well as any news about her grandchildren. Around 7:10 P.M., I would say, *"Well, it's about time for me to go home and get some dinner."*

"You call this a visit?" she would ask, using a tone she had perfected to induce maximum guilt.

"Ma, I leave at the exact same time every night!" I would respond in exasperation. She would just shrug.

At the time of my mother's death, in April of 1996, I was in Washington, D. C., giving the plenary lecture at the annual Federation of American Societies for Experimental Biology meeting. Lynn was with me and received the call from the nursing home just before I took the stage. Lynn let me give my talk, then told me afterward that my mother had passed. We flew home to Durham, had a service for my mom, then flew to New York City to bury my mother next to my father.

◆

With my mother's death from cardiac complications and my own ongoing recovery from quadruple bypass surgery, my family history of heart trouble was at the forefront of my mind in the mid-1990s. Coincidentally, or perhaps not so coincidentally, the research in my lab in this era veered toward animal models of cardiac disease. For most of my career to that point, I had been mainly focused on basic research questions: Do receptors exist? How do receptors work? These types of studies had tangential connections to human disease, insofar as receptors are important drug targets, but the research itself was very basic in nature. This pure focus on basic research changed, though, when Carmelo Milano joined my lab.

Carmelo was part of the cardiothoracic surgery residency program at Duke run by David Sabiston. As mentioned in an earlier chapter, Sabiston was one of the most distinguished cardiac surgeons in the world at that time, and the residency program he established became known as the "Decade with Dave." During this ten-year training program, residents would take an exam each year to test their knowledge of everything having to do with surgery. The expectation was that residents would get progressively better at this exam as they moved through the program, with first-year residents scoring fairly low, fourth-year residents showing improvement, and tenth-year residents scoring the highest. However, during Carmelo's first year in the program, he scored higher on this exam than any of the tenth-year residents, and in fact scored higher on the exam than any resident had ever scored in the history of the program. Carmelo carried himself with a surgeon's demeanor—self-assured, steady as a rock—and Sabiston was convinced he was one of the most exceptional surgery residents to ever train at Duke.

Given Sabiston's high opinion of Carmelo's abilities, he wanted to push Carmelo to expand his horizons. During the "Decade with Dave," residents were expected to conduct two years of research. Most residents chose to conduct their research in cardiac physiology labs, staying close to their clinical interests. However, Sabiston pushed Carmelo to get out of his comfort zone and join my lab, with the goal of shooting for the moon during his two-year research stint.

Carmelo knew nothing about molecular biology when he started. I initially assigned him a project to see if he could make a "transgenic" mouse that would overexpress the alpha-1B adrenergic receptor in certain tissues to see if this led to cancer. After a few months Carmelo asked to meet with me one day and sheepishly admitted that he would be much happier if he could work on something more directly relevant to the heart. I told him that some other folks in the lab had accidentally discovered a way to make adrenergic receptors highly active even in the absence of adrenaline. Such receptors are called "constitutively active,"[1] and I was curious to see what might happen if we expressed such constitutively active beta receptors in the heart.

At this time, I knew very little about the recently developed transgenic techniques that would be required to express an unnatural receptor in the heart of a mouse. I really didn't have much advice to offer Carmelo for this project other than a vague vision of what we hoped to achieve. However, Carmelo was undaunted by the lab's lack of expertise in this area; he read the literature for a few days, talked to some experts on campus, and devised a strategy. Amazingly, in just a few months, Carmelo successfully generated a mouse line expressing overactive beta receptors in their hearts.

Following Carmelo's technical success, our next problem was how to actually study these mice. As a clinician, I had performed lots of cardiac studies on humans, but how do you study cardiac physiology in a mouse? I had absolutely no idea. Carmelo surveyed the literature and told me there was a group at the University of California San Diego who had developed cutting-edge techniques for performing cardiac studies on mice. This group was led by a renowned senior cardiac physiologist named John Ross, but the key player was a junior faculty member named Howard Rockman. One day, I called Rockman out of the blue to see if he might be interested in collaborating. He answered his office phone and I introduced myself.

"Hello, Dr. Rockman? This is Bob Lefkowitz." The next thing I heard was a loud crash. A few seconds later, Rockman was back on the line, saying, *"Sorry about that, Dr. Lefkowitz!"* Rockman would later tell me that he was so excited when he heard my voice that he literally dropped the phone. It was a collaboration made in heaven: we were excited to work with Rockman because of his expertise with cardiac studies in mice, and he was excited to work with us because of our expertise with receptors.

We sent Carmelo's mice to Rockman and right away the findings were stunning. The cardiac output of the transgenic mice was jaw dropping: their hearts beat much faster and harder than the hearts of normal mice. This made sense because these transgenic hearts were now loaded with receptors that no longer needed adrenaline for stimulation, so it was like the hearts were soaked in adrenaline all the time. However, subsequent studies yielded a mystery: the receptors that were expressed by these transgenic mice did not exhibit the properties we expected from overactive beta-2 adrenergic receptors. Further analysis revealed that the transgenic mice actually expressed normal beta-2 receptors, and we eventually figured out that somebody in the lab had accidentally given Carmelo normal beta-2 receptor DNA rather than mutant receptor DNA when he was first creating the transgenic animals. Thus, Carmelo had ended up making mice that had regular beta-2 receptors in their hearts but at a density of receptors that was three hundred times the normal level, resulting in the massive increase in cardiac output.

The interesting findings with these mice were all the more serendipitous because when Carmelo subsequently created a line of mice that actually *did* express the overactive mutant beta-2 receptors in the heart, the results were much less exciting. In fact, these mice seemed completely normal in virtually all respects, with the levels of beta receptors in their heart tissue being almost completely the same as regular mice. We eventually figured out that cardiac cells can sense the overactive receptors as being abnormal and suppress their expression, presumably as a mechanism to protect the heart. In fact, we found that the only way to even detect expression of the overactive receptors was to treat the mice with beta blockers, which silenced the overactive receptors and allowed them to finally be observed.[2]

In subsequent studies, Carmelo created a line of mice that overexpressed constitutively active alpha-1B adrenergic receptors in cardiac tissue. These mice exhibited many of the features seen in human patients with cardiac hypertrophy, a pathological overgrowth of heart tissue. In this way, we accidentally created a useful model for studying cardiac hypertrophy. In related studies, Wally Koch, a postdoctoral fellow in my lab, worked with Carmelo to create lines of mice marked by cardiac expression of either beta-adrenergic receptor kinase (the enzyme that phosphorylates and regulates beta receptors) or pieces of this kinase. Some of these lines of mice exhibited features of human patients suffering from chronic heart failure, so these mice also proved to be useful cardiac disease models.[3]

Cardiac disease had killed both my father and mother, and almost killed me before I had a chance to meet my first grandchild. These translational studies that my lab pursued in the 1990s were satisfying because it felt good to "punch back" against cardiac disease in some way and create models that might lead to new cardiac therapies down the road. I still viewed myself as a basic researcher, but felt excited to make headway in fighting back against the disease that had wreaked such havoc on my family over the years.

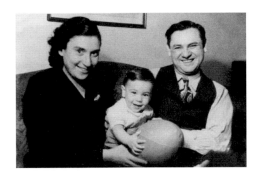

ABOVE: I was born in 1943 to Max and Rose Lefkowitz. As an only child, I had the full focus of my parents' attention, for better and/or worse. BELOW: My childhood dream was to be the next Mickey Mantle, but my complete lack of hitting, fielding, and running ability diverted me into medicine.

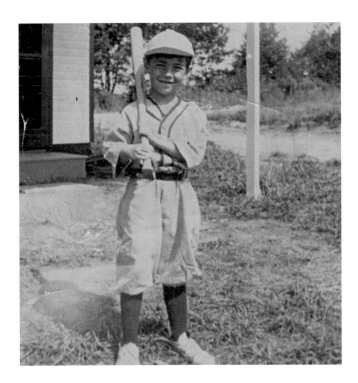

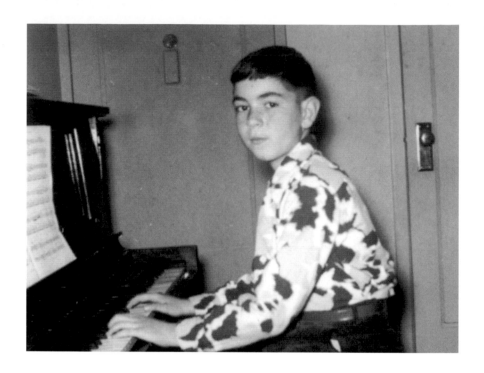

ABOVE: I gained discipline from piano lessons, which I hated but were strictly enforced by my mother. BELOW: The 1950s were an era in which muscle men were worshipped, so during high school my buddies and I tirelessly pumped iron.

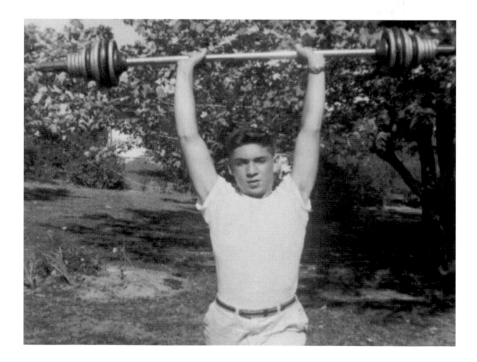

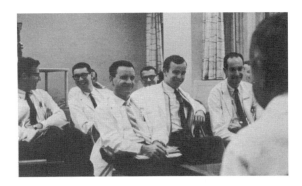

ABOVE: In medical school, one of my classmates was future Nobel Laureate and NIH Director Harold Varmus (far left). In this photo, I'm second from the left, sharing a laugh with Harold. BELOW: At my graduation from Columbia medical school, I smiled for a photo with my parents but was feeling stressed about the "doctor draft" that might send me to Vietnam. Touchingly, my father told me that it was "the proudest day of his life."

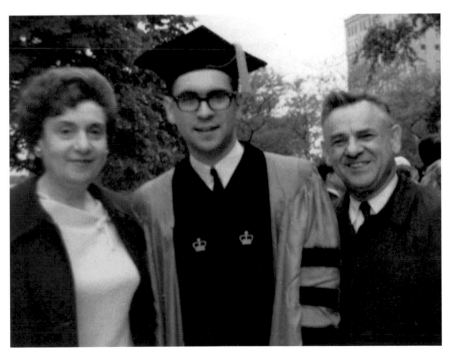

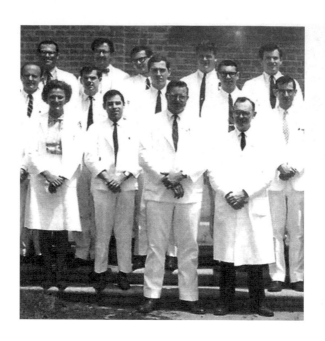

ABOVE: This photo of the house staff of the Columbia Presbyterian Medical Center in 1967 includes Harold Varmus (top row, second from left) and myself (second row, second from right) in addition to our hulking Chief Resident Bill Lovejoy (front row on the left, center of photo), a former All-American football player at Yale who ran a tight ship. BELOW: As a member of the "Yellow Berets," I was able to serve my country while staying stateside rather than heading to Vietnam. In this 1968 U.S. Public Health Service photo of the staff of the National Institute of Arthritis and Metabolic Diseases (as it was then known), I'm in the third row, second from the left, and joined by two fellow Yellow Berets who would later go on to win Nobel Prizes: Harold Varmus (top row, third from left) and Mike Brown (second row, second from left).

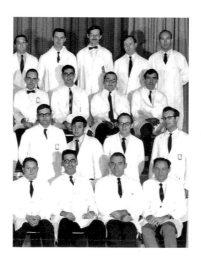

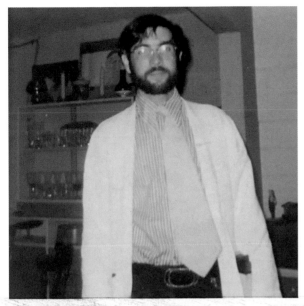

During my senior residency and cardiology fellowship at Massachusetts General Hospital, I missed research and began sneaking into the lab to do experiments when I was supposed to be completing my clinical rotations. The group photo shown below is the MGH residency class of 1970–71; I am in the top row, second from the right.

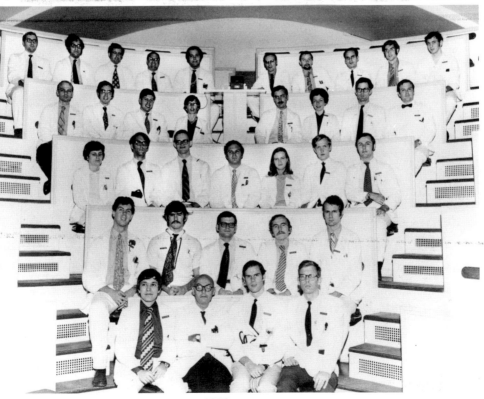

1970

FIRST ROW	R. Genteler, A. Leaf, J. Franklin, C. Hopkins
SECOND ROW	E. Hoffer, P. Simpson, G. McGuffin, T. Murray, L. Mallette
THIRD ROW	N. Stead, W. Ricks, L. Bennion, J. Borer, R. Stevens, R Matta, R. Fisher
FOURTH ROW	R. Gibson, S. Howell, D. Krogstad, J. Marmor, L. Axelrad, A. Baker, P. Mogielnicki, J. Mull
FIFTH ROW	R. Re, P. Cohen, W. Seaman, M. Pohl, R. Marier, G. Khoury, J. Anderson, D. Scott, R. Lefkowitz, L. Bercovitch

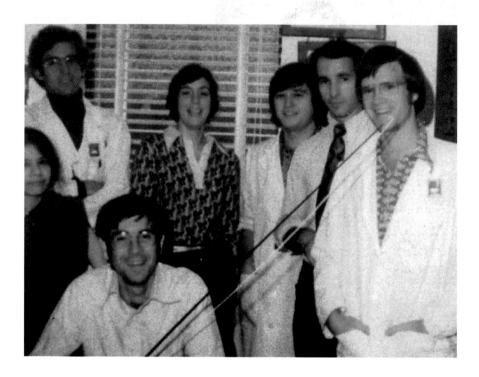

ABOVE: As a new faculty member setting up my lab at Duke in the mid 1970s, my hiring strategy was simple: take anyone who walked in the door. Fortunately, I happened to be joined by a collection of exceptionally talented young scientists, including (standing from left to right) post-doc Chobi Mukherjee, medical student John Mickey, post-doc Lee Limbird, post-doc Marc Caron, cardiology fellow Wayne Alexander, and MD/PhD student Rusty Williams. BELOW: While my lab at Duke was expanding, my family at home was growing as well. This photo from the late 1970s shows Arna and me with our kids (from left to right) Cheryl, Larry (Noah), Mara, Joshua (in my arms), and David.

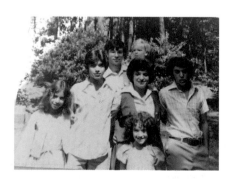

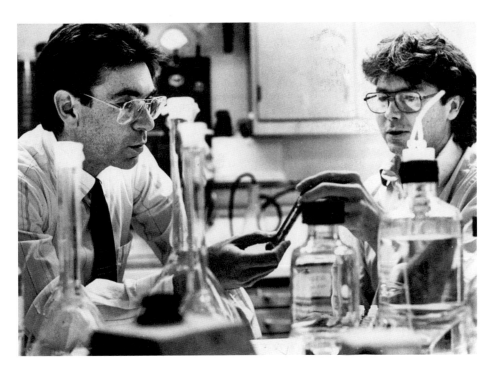

ABOVE: This photo from the early 1980s captures me doing something I love: schmoozing in the lab with my trainees. In this case, I'm deep in conversation with my post-doc John Regan. During this era, a sign was mysteriously affixed to my office door pronouncing me the "Sultan of Schmooze." BELOW: In the mid-1980s, the receptor cloning team in my lab was working hard and needed a break, so I rewarded them with a limo ride to lunch at the restaurant of their choice. They ended up taking the limo to the drive-through window at McDonald's. Shown here from left to right are Henrik Dohlman, Brian Kobilka, Tong-Sun Kobilka, Debbie Frielle, Tom Frielle, and Mark Bolanowski.

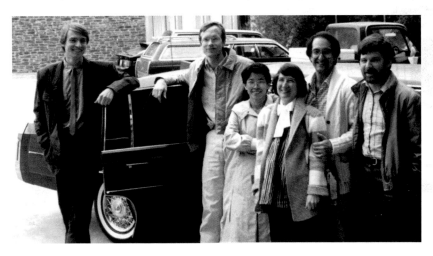

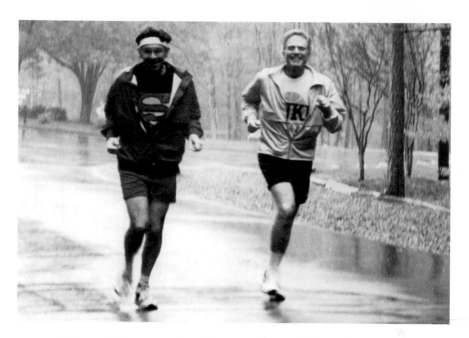

ABOVE: Before and after my quadruple bypass surgery, Ralph Snyderman was my main running partner as well as my scientific collaborator, confidante, and friend. BELOW LEFT: In the 1990s, my good friend Tony Fauci and I served together for a decade on the council of the Association of American Physicians (AAP). In this photo from an AAP council meeting, I'm the one speaking and Tony is to my right. BELOW RIGHT: During a break from a scientific meeting in Scotland in 1992, I went for a walk with Al Gilman and we came across a street called "Rotten Row." Al immediately suggested that this seemed a fitting locale for two dirty rotten scoundrels like us, so we stopped for a photo. Gilman and I were ferocious competitors in the 1970s and 1980s, but by the 1990s we had developed a strong mutual respect and friendship.

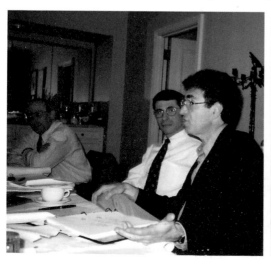

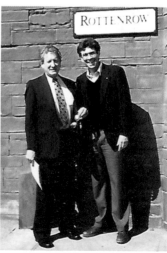

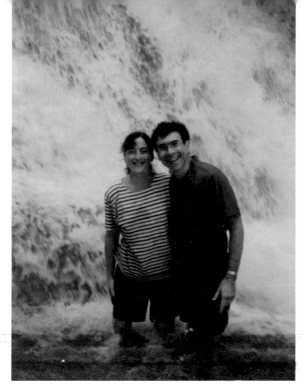

TOP: In both my recovery from quadruple bypass surgery and my emotional recovery following my divorce, my second wife Lynn was an absolute rock for me.

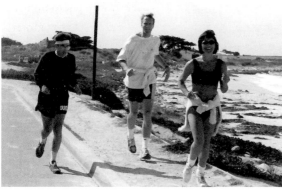

CENTER: Mentoring is a job for life. In this photo taken during a break from a scientific meeting in California in the late 1990s, I am doing my best to keep up with two former trainees, Brian Kobilka and Sheila Collins, who by that time were both faculty members directing their own labs.

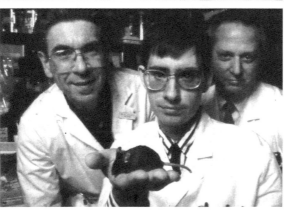

BOTTOM: An exciting new direction for the lab in the 1990's was the creation of transgenic mice with altered adrenergic receptor activity. Shown here is a newspaper photo from 1994 featuring one of these transgenic mice. Carmelo Milano is holding the mouse, flanked by Lee Allen (right) and me. *Courtesy of* The Herald Sun.

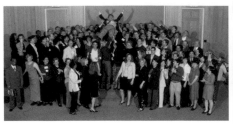
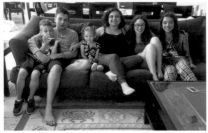

ABOVE LEFT: For my 60th birthday in 2003, more than a hundred alumni from my lab returned to Duke for a two-day celebration and roast. We took a group photo in which I fulfilled a lifelong dream of crowdsurfing on a mosh pit, trusting my trainees not to drop me. ABOVE RIGHT: In addition to having a large and loving scientific family, I am also blessed with a large and loving biological family. Like every grandparent, I believe that all of my grandchildren are wonderful, adorable, and worthy of being celebrated in endless photos. From left to right in this pic are: Ethan Lefkowitz, Jonah Herbsman, Emmy Lefkowitz, Maya Herbsman, Madeleine Lefkowitz, and Samantha Lefkowitz. BELOW: The key to a successful career in research is to have great collaborators. My most prolific collaborator has been Marc Caron, with whom I have published more than 250 papers. There's just something about Marc that makes me smile, as shown here.

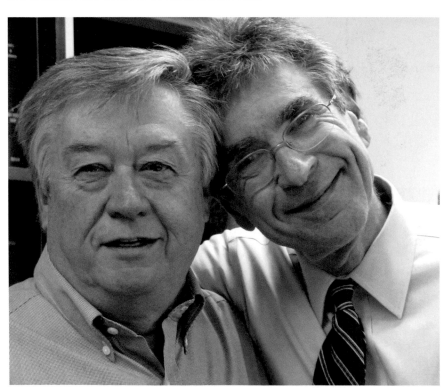

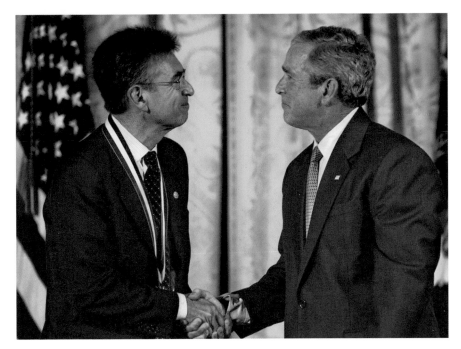

ABOVE: In 2008, I was honored to receive the National Medal of Science from President George W. Bush. I would have preferred to receive the award a few months later when Barack Obama was in the White House, but I had to admit that President Bush was very funny and charming in person. BELOW: This photo of me in my office at Duke captures a pose that all of my trainees will undoubtedly find familiar: feet up on the desk, smile on my face, exulting over the latest data.

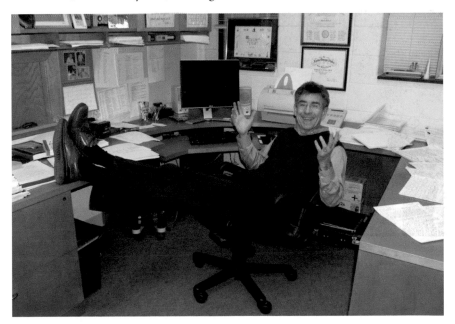

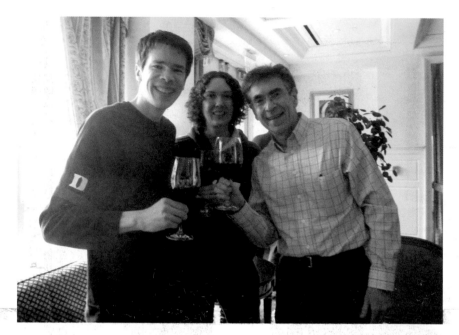

ABOVE: My former trainee (and the co-author of this book) Randy Hall and his wife Liberty are shown here enjoying a pre-game drink with me at the Washington Duke Inn before heading to a Duke basketball game in 2011. BELOW LEFT: After I received word in October 2012 that I won the Nobel Prize, I was honored in a pre-season ceremony at Cameron Indoor Stadium. BELOW RIGHT: One of the perks of the ceremony at Cameron was getting to spend time with Coach K and all the guys on the Duke basketball team.

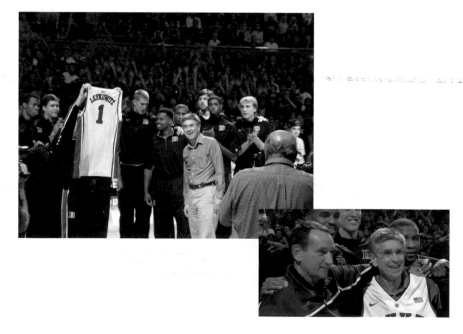

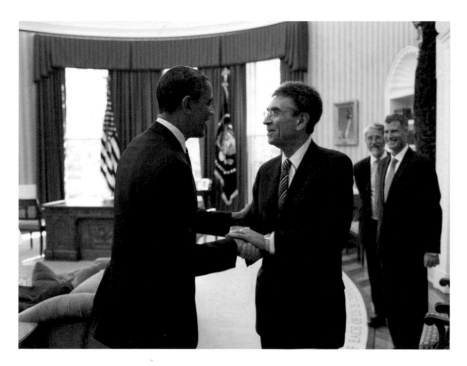

ABOVE: Before heading to Stockholm for the Nobel festivities, I visited the White House (along with the other American Laureates that year) for an enjoyable chat with President Obama. BELOW: It was a great delight to share the Nobel Prize with a former trainee. This photo of Brian Kobilka and me was taken just a few moments after we finished our Nobel Lectures. *Photo by Roger Sunahara.*

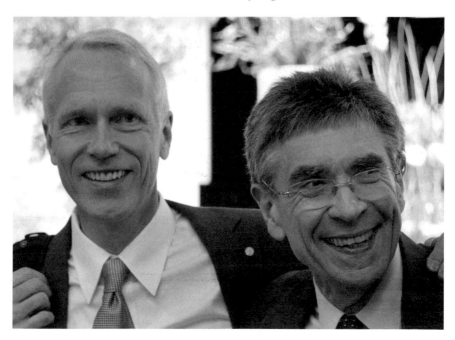

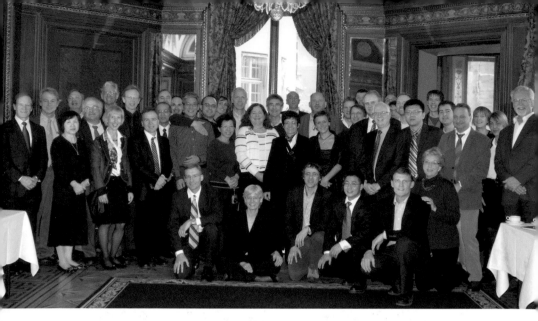

ABOVE: Brian and I were joined by numerous alumni from our labs for the Nobel festivities. Here we are celebrating at a hugely enjoyable reception with our trainees, colleagues, and collaborators at the Grand Hotel on the day before the Nobel Ceremony and Banquet. Science is a team sport, so it was fun to celebrate as a team. BELOW: It was also wonderful to share the Nobel festivities with my family. Shown here from left to right are: Joshua Lefkowitz, David Lefkowitz, his wife Michelle, Lynn Lefkowitz, Me, Mara Lefkowitz Mack, Cheryl Herbsman, Mara's boyfriend (now husband) Eric Mack, Maya Herbsman, Jonah Herbsman, Wade McCollum (Noah's husband), Oded Herbsman (Cheryl's husband), Noah Jordan, and my cousin Ellen Danziger. *Copyright ©Nobel Media, photo by Alexander Mahmoud.*

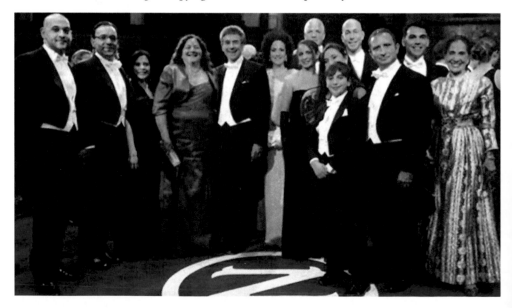

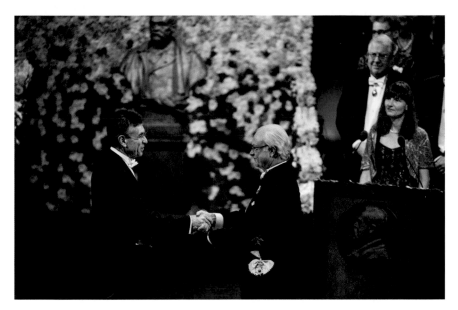

ABOVE: There is no shortage of pomp and circumstance during the Nobel festivities. This is the moment when I received the Nobel Medal from King Carl XVI Gustaf. *Copyright © Nobel Media, photo by Alex Ljungdahl.* BELOW: A year after winning the Nobel Prize, I was invited to throw out the ceremonial first pitch at a Durham Bulls baseball game. This photo shows the pre-game ceremony before the first pitch featuring Mayor of Durham Bill Bell (far right), President of the Duke Health System Victor Dzau, and the Bulls's mascot Wool E. Bull. Several minutes later, I threw a strike for the game's first pitch.

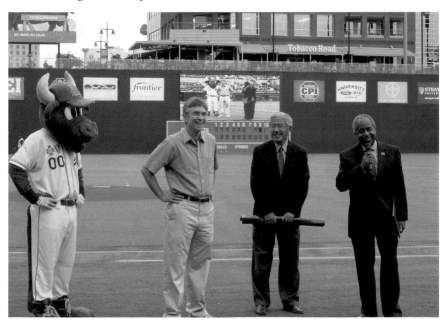

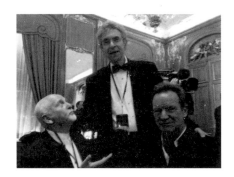

ABOVE: At the Academy of Achievement Summit in London in 2017, Peter Gabriel (far left) and Sting knelt before me in a show of faux adulation meant to impress my son David, who works in the music industry. BELOW: No matter what other adventures are on offer, my favorite place to be is still in the lab, schmoozing with my trainees, analyzing data, and dreaming up future experiments. In this photo, I'm sketching out a plan of action with medical student Erin Bressler.

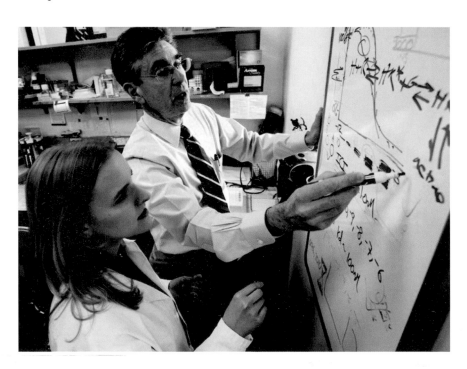

EIGHTEEN

Jeopardy!

I was sitting down to dinner with my wife Lynn when my Uncle Henry called, breathless with excitement.

"Bobby! Bobby, I'm so proud of you. I can't even believe it. Your name was an answer on *Jeopardy!*"

I tried to interject something, but the words just kept pouring out of Uncle Henry's mouth in a torrent.

"It was something about sperm! Like, how does the sperm sense the egg? Oh Bobby, I'm just so proud of you. When you make it to Scotland, I'm coming with you."

"Scotland? Why would I be going to Scotland?" I asked.

"You know, when you win that big prize," he replied.

"Do you mean Stockholm?"

"Scotland, Stockholm, what's the difference? I know you're going to win it soon. If your name is being mentioned on *Jeopardy!*, you must be getting close."

Uncle Henry was calling from New York City, where he obsessively watched the game show *Jeopardy!* every evening at 6:00 P.M. In Durham, North Carolina, *Jeopardy!* didn't air until 6:30 P.M., so Lynn and I turned on the TV and watched *Jeopardy!* during dinner. Sure enough, halfway through the first round, the $200 question in the category "Science News" was: *"In 1995 Dr. Robert Lefkowitz discovered sperm uses this sense to track down the egg."* The contestant correctly responded, *"What is smell?"*

Given the status of *Jeopardy!* as the premier TV game show in the USA, many people would view it as the culmination of a lifelong dream to have their name featured in a *Jeopardy!* answer. In my case, I had finally made it onto *Jeopardy!*, but with a major caveat: I was being credited with a discovery that I didn't actually make.

I have never conducted research on sperm motility. Indeed, despite the fact that I am a father of five, I must confess that I know very little about sperm. So how did it happen that my name ended up associated with a question about sperm on the *Jeopardy!* episode that aired on October 7, 1996? The answer to that question requires a flashback to a year and a half earlier.

In early 1995, a science writers' conference was held at Duke. This annual event changed location each year, but the format was the same: several dozen prominent science writers would convene and listen to talks from eminent scientists to learn about the latest cutting-edge research in different fields. Given that the 1995 edition of this event was held at Duke, I was invited to participate and talk about my lab's work on the fundamental biology of G protein–coupled receptors. After my presentation, one of the reporters asked, *"Is there anything else going on in your field that we should know about?"* I replied that G protein–coupled receptors do a lot more than just mediate responses to adrenaline and other hormones. For example, there are specialized odorant receptors in the nose that mediate the sense of smell. Moreover, a recent report from a group in Belgium had even shown that several of these odorant receptors are found in sperm, where they may play a role helping the sperm to find the egg.

The next morning after this science writers' conference, I received a call from my son David, who was living in San Francisco at the time.

"Hey, Dad, I didn't know you were working on sperm," David said.

"What are you talking about?" I asked.

"There's an article in the *San Francisco Chronicle* this morning about how you discovered that sperm use their sense of smell to find the egg," David continued. "It sounds really interesting."

I thanked David for letting me know and told him that there had been a mistake I needed to correct. Unfortunately, as soon as I hung up from talking to David, I began to get other calls from various friends and colleagues asking about my new research interest in sperm. It turned out that the article David had seen in the San Francisco paper was written by a reporter from the Associated Press. Thus, this article had run in hundreds of newspapers around the world in addition to running in the *Chronicle*.

When I'd agreed to speak at the science writers' conference, I had been told that no stories would be published without approval from the scientists who gave the talks. However, I had not been contacted by the reporter from the Associated Press prior to publication of the sperm article. This article had just gone straight to press crediting me with the discovery about odorant receptors in sperm.

Needless to say, I was mortified: I didn't want the researchers in Belgium to think that I was trying to take credit for their discovery. The first thing I did was call the Associated Press to set the record straight. They put out a clarification, but as with most clarifications, very few people saw it. Lots of people read the original article, which received incredible media attention, but very few people read the subsequent clarification in which I made clear I was talking about someone else's work. The second thing I did was call Gilbert Vassart, the Belgian scientist who was the senior author of the original article about odorant receptors in sperm.[1] I told Vassart the story about the science writers' conference and how I had given his group appropriate credit for the work, but somehow the journalist had simply gotten it wrong. Vassart was very understanding and thought the whole story was funny.

After contacting both the Associated Press and the Belgian group, I thought the story was over. However, it turned out that the story was just beginning. Someone from the *Jeopardy!* "clue crew" found the original article about a year after its publication but failed to find the clarification. And that was how my name ended up in a *Jeopardy!* question about sperm.

It wasn't just my Uncle Henry who saw my name mentioned on *Jeopardy!* that October evening in 1996. In the days that followed, I received numerous calls and emails from various family members, friends, and colleagues who had either seen the *Jeopardy!* show or heard about it. For the first few callers, I tried to explain the whole story, including the science writers' conference, the confusion over my comment about the Belgian group's work, et cetera. However, it took a huge effort to tell this story over and over again to every single person who called. Thus, after a few calls, I just began accepting all the congratulations without trying to explain.

"Yes indeed, it was exciting to see my name mentioned on *Jeopardy!* Yes, I know it may seem surprising that the question was about sperm, but research always takes you in unexpected directions."

After the hullabaloo over the *Jeopardy!* question died down, I figured that my career as a sperm expert was finally over. Sadly, I was mistaken. In the years that followed, I received countless random calls and emails relating to this episode. One memorable call, several years after the *Jeopardy!* episode, was from a young lady who was a writer for *Flare*, a women's fashion magazine in Canada that's like a Canadian version of *Cosmopolitan.*

"Dr. Lefkowitz, we're putting together our annual gynecology update issue," said the journalist. "And we're hoping to get a quote from you about your research on sperm and the development of a male contraceptive."

I was tempted to say something crazy, just to give this journalist a juicy quote that would keep my legend as a sperm authority alive for another few decades. However, common sense kicked in and I told the journalist that she should actually talk with Gilbert Vassart in Belgium if she wanted to get an update on the latest research on chemical sensing by sperm.

I have the greatest respect for journalists, who have the difficult job of conveying complex information to the public. At the same time, I have found that it can be hazardous as a scientist to communicate with journalists. Like most scientists, I strive hard to make my research sound as interesting as possible when I write grant applications, which are aimed at convincing other scientists that the work is important enough to get funded. When I communicate with journalists, though, I have found that I need to take the opposite approach: rather than promoting my research, I need to undersell it and downplay it, because otherwise the journalist will end up making grandiose claims about the work that go far beyond what the research has actually shown.

Another example of overzealous journalism was the time I was credited with solving the mystery of why hair turns gray. Some years after the *Jeopardy!* episode, my lab published a paper in *Nature* about how beta-2 adrenergic receptors mediate stress responses that lead to DNA damage.[2] At the request of the journal, I talked to a small group of journalists to explain this work and tried to give examples of the deleterious effects of stress, briefly mentioning the graying of hair as one example. The study that my lab had published in *Nature* had nothing to do with gray hair, but rather was focused on basic cellular responses to stress. However, after I mentioned gray hair to the journalists, the media coverage of this work somehow became a narrative that was focused entirely on my lab's dramatic efforts to combat gray hair.

Given the fact that I've been incorrectly portrayed in the media as both a sperm expert and gray hair guru, you might think that I would just stop talking to journalists. In truth, though, I think it's very important for scientists to convey to the public the relevance of their research findings, because so much research is funded by taxpayer dollars. The public needs to know how their tax dollars are being spent, so it's crucial for scientists to take the time to engage and explain. At the same time, it's very important for scientists to avoid overhyping their work or overpromising potential benefits to the public. This is especially critical because there are politicians who are antiscience and seek to use any blatant overpromising as a cudgel to bash science and scientists. Thus, given the natural inclination of journalists to hype their articles, scientists actually need to *undersell* their research as much as possible when talking to the media, pointing out all the caveats, even though such efforts at understatement can often feel counterintuitive.

Another forum in which I've had extensive interactions with the media has been as the leader of scholarly societies. I've had the pleasure of being elected president of both the American Society for Clinical Investigation (ASCI) and the Association of American Physicians (AAP). When I gave my ASCI presidential address in 1988, I focused on research ethics, which was a timely topic because there had been several newsworthy cases of scientific fraud in the preceding years. During my address, I talked about the various ways that scientists can fool themselves, referencing the classic book *On Bullshit* by Harry Frankfurt in making the point that scientists need to be careful not to bullshit themselves or others. When I finished my talk, I took my seat next to Joe Goldstein, a former ASCI president and good friend of mine since our days together as Yellow Berets at the NIH.

"Nice talk," said Joe. "But why did you have to say 'bullshit' so many times?"

"How many times did I say it?" I asked. Joe looked directly into my eyes.

"Ten."

When I got back to my hotel room at the end of the evening, I checked the text of my remarks and counted the number of times I had said "bullshit."[3] It was exactly ten. My friend Joe was a proper gentleman who clearly didn't appreciate cursing in public, and I imagined him tensing up and counting every time I had said "bullshit" in my lecture. Hopefully my anti-bullshit message got across even if my language offended some sensibilities during that address.

Some years later, in 2001, I served as president of the AAP during a very challenging time for the society. Membership in the AAP had been declining throughout the 1990s, due in part to an unfortunate trend away from physicians conducting research. I was concerned about this trend, as was Tony Fauci, my friend and fellow Yellow Beret who had served as the society's president the previous year. Tony and I had been elected to the AAP Council in consecutive years a decade earlier, knowing that we would each serve as president in 2000 and 2001, respectively. At one point in the mid-1990s, we graphed the decline in attendance to the annual AAP meeting, and depending on how the line was drawn it looked like it might hit zero around the turn of the millennium. Tony and I kidded each other about which of us would be the first president to preside over an annual AAP meeting with nobody in attendance. Fortunately, we were able to take measures to boost membership and keep the society vibrant, which meant that neither of us had to give a presidential address to an empty room.

Given that my presidential address to the AAP came in 2001, I arranged with the audiovisual team to open my lecture in dramatic fashion. Just as I took the stage for my address, the room went completely dark and the theme from *2001: A Space Odyssey* began pulsating through the ballroom. The screen then lit up with an image of my face in an astronaut's helmet, floating in space. After a minute, the music stopped, the lights came back on, and the crowd stood as one to applaud the spectacle.

"Well, maybe I should just sit down now, since I already received my standing ovation," I said before beginning my remarks.

My AAP address focused on the importance of exposing physicians to research.[4] I told the story of a colleague of mine from Duke, Bill Hall, who took up jogging in his late thirties as part of an effort to stop smoking. It soon became apparent that Bill possessed an uncommon gift for distance running. With limited training, he rapidly became faster than all of his more experienced training partners and began winning local races. After just a couple of years of training, he won the USA men's masters marathon championship at the age of forty with a time of 2:21, which qualified him for the USA Olympic Trials marathon. None of this would've happened, of course, if Bill hadn't been exposed to running in his thirties and realized this incredible gift he possessed.

I told this story during my AAP presidential address because I believe there are many physicians who could be great researchers, but will never realize this fact unless they are exposed to research. Look at my own career as an example: I was not exposed to research until I serendipitously ended up at the NIH in fulfillment of my draft obligation during the Vietnam War. Once I began doing research, I fell in love with it and realized I possessed some aptitude in this area. I was an accidental scientist, and it was only through a well-designed (and taxpayer-funded) program—the Public Health Service Commissioned Corps—that I became exposed to research.

At Duke, we require all third-year medical students to conduct a year of research, and almost all of the fellowship and residency programs at Duke also require a year or two of research. However, many medical schools do not have such requirements to expose their trainees to research. In my mind, that's a shame. Who knows how many physicians are out there with untapped potential to make game-changing discoveries to promote human health? It was for this reason that I made exposure of physicians to research a central theme of my AAP presidency. I wanted to make the point that there are many current and future physicians who could become accidental scientists like me if given the opportunity to experience the joy that comes from doing research and making discoveries.

In spite of the accidental nature of my research career, and also in spite of the jeopardy I've sometimes found myself in while trying to convey the importance of my lab's research to the public, word did eventually get around regarding my lab's contributions to understanding receptors, and I began to win some major awards. As my mother would've said, they weren't the Nobel Prize, but nonetheless, I was very honored to receive such recognition. Moreover, traveling the globe to receive these awards resulted in a number of adventures (and misadventures) that kept my adrenaline pumping.

NINETEEN

The International Scientific Prize Circuit

My name was announced over the loudspeaker. As the echoes reverberated throughout the arena, I received my cue from a guy in a headset and began my journey down the red carpet.

I was about to receive the Shaw Prize, often referred to as the "Nobel of the East." The Shaw Prize was bankrolled by Run Run Shaw, the billionaire who had launched the Hong Kong movie industry. The venue for the awards ceremony was the cavernous Grand Hall of the Hong Kong Convention and Exhibition Centre, and my walk down the red carpet to the stage went past a large throng of cheering attendees. It seemed to take forever.

The stage was flanked by two massive jumbotrons on which I could see myself walking. As I watched my own image, I noticed that my right shoulder looked lower than my left. I have always been self-conscious about my posture: when I was growing up, my mother persistently chastised me for poor posture, claiming my shoulders weren't even because I carried my book bag solely on one side. When I saw my uneven shoulders on the jumbotron, I tried to rearrange myself but ended up overcorrecting. Not only did I look awkward, but now my left shoulder was much lower than my right. I recorrected again but still looked off-kilter as I made it to the stage. When I sat down later next to Lynn, she leaned over with a whispered question.

"What in the *world* were you doing with your shoulders?"

Presiding over the ceremony was Run Run Shaw, who looked clinically dead. With all due respect, he was 100 years old, but he looked like he'd been embalmed. He sat motionless throughout the entire ceremony while citations were read describing my research as well as the work of the other Shaw Prize recipients in Astronomy and Mathematical Sciences (my prize was for Life Sciences and Medicine). When the ceremony was over, the other winners and I were invited to pose for photographs around Mr. Shaw, who remained as inert as a wax figure. I began to feel somewhat concerned, as I hadn't seen him move at all during the entire proceedings. My training as a clinician kicked in and I eyeballed him carefully for several minutes to discern if he was breathing. Finally, in a sloth-like manner, Mr. Shaw slowly rotated his head and met my gaze, his face wrinkling into a wry smile. I smiled back, feeling relieved and thinking to myself how much I would love to still be hosting gala events at 100 years old.

The Shaw Prize came with a $1 million honorarium, and we were told that the money would be wired into our bank accounts the morning after the ceremony. Lynn and I were curious to see if the transfer would actually occur as scheduled. Moreover, we were interested to see what our bank account would look like after the transfer. The money would be transferred in Hong Kong dollars; with an exchange rate of 8:1 at that time, this meant we would supposedly see $8 million in our account, an eye-popping sum regardless of exchange rate. Indeed, we checked our balance at the hotel ATM machine and saw a balance in excess of $8 million. Lynn insisted I take a photo of the screen because it was such an impressive-looking number.

We spent that day sightseeing around Hong Kong, and then spent the next day after that traveling back to the USA. We landed in Washington, D. C., where we had another event to attend because I was scheduled to receive an honorary award from the Heart Failure Society of America. After spending the night at a hotel, we got up the next morning and were curious to see how our bank account now looked in American dollars. As we strolled to the hotel restaurant for breakfast, we stopped to check our balance at an ATM in the lobby and saw a balance of $8,950. Befuddled, I took out the card, pressed "reset" and tried again but got the same result: $8,950. What happened to the million dollars? Suddenly, I was in a panic. I told Lynn we needed to call our bank's twenty-four-hour customer service number to figure out what the problem was.

"Yes, let's call them after breakfast," Lynn suggested, always the calm and reasonable one.

"The hell with breakfast," I replied. "We just lost a million dollars. I want to know what's going on."

We went straight back up to our room, and I called the bank. After explaining the situation to several different people, I was finally routed to a supervisor who said, *"Ah yes, Dr. Lefkowitz, someone should have told you that our ATM machines don't show digits beyond six digits. So your actual balance in that account is $1,008,950, but it just doesn't show up on the ATM."* I breathed a huge sigh of relief and headed back downstairs with Lynn to finally enjoy some breakfast.

Some months after I received the Shaw Prize, I got a call in my office from someone claiming to be the science advisor to the president of the United States. I was skeptical at first, but the guy sounded legit, so I kept talking to him. He said that I was going to receive the National Medal of Science, the highest honor that the United States government confers on scientists, in a special ceremony with the president at the White House. This call came in September 2008, when it was increasingly obvious that Barack Obama was going to win the November election to become the next president. As an admirer of Obama, I was excited at the prospect of getting the chance to meet him. However, I realized that even if Obama won the election, he wouldn't actually become president until January. With some trepidation, I queried the science advisor about when exactly the ceremony would take place, hoping that it might still be several months away.

"Oh, the ceremony will be in just a few weeks, on September 29," the science adviser said. I was crestfallen as I realized that I would have to receive the Medal of Science from George W. Bush, a president I definitely did not admire.

I showed up at the White House on the specified date with a small entourage consisting of Lynn, my kids, several other family members, some folks from my laboratory staff, plus Dick Brodhead, the president of Duke. We went through a rigorous security check and were led to the East Room, where there was a lovely ceremony. The other winner in Biology that year was Bert O'Malley from Baylor, who was best known for studying nuclear hormone receptors (i.e., receptors found in the nucleus of the cell). Bush had a well-known quirk of pronouncing the word "nuclear" as "nu-cu-lar," and I was looking forward to hearing him repeatedly mispronouncing the word while reading O'Malley's citation. However, it turned out that a presidential spokesperson read the citations for each scholar, and the only job of the president was to place the medals around our necks. I suspected that Bush's staff didn't want to risk having him stumble through all the big science words in the text.

After the ceremony, the winners had fifteen minutes or so to chat with the president as a small group. I truly disliked President Bush for many of his policies, but I must confess that in person I found him delightful. He was charming, funny, and an absolute pleasure to be around. Somehow we ended up talking about our spouses, and the love he expressed for his wife, Laura, was very touching. Considering all the things going wrong in Bush's presidency at that time, including the crashing economy and unpopular war in Iraq, I was impressed with Bush's ability to work a room and make everyone smile.

Around this same time, I was fortunate enough to win a couple of European science prizes. The first was several years earlier when I won the Lefoulon-Delalande Foundation Grand Prize for Science, a French award that came with a cash prize of 500,000 euros. I won this prize at the best time possible, just as the US dollar was crashing against the euro. After I was publicly announced as the winner, I had to wait several months to actually receive the award, and the euros, at a ceremony in Paris. During that time, the value of the prize in US dollars kept going up and up. I don't normally cheer for the US dollar to fall, but during these few months I sometimes caught myself fist-pumping while watching the news and hearing reports that the dollar had another rough day against the euro.

While attending the ceremony in Paris, Lynn and I stayed at a swanky hotel called the George V ("George cinq"). One evening when we were heading out to dinner, we rode down the hotel's preposterously tiny elevator to the lobby and walked toward the front doors. Just as we were about to exit, we walked past Mick Jagger, who was strutting in with a tall, elegant woman. I saw that they were headed for the elevator we had come out of a minute earlier. I turned to Lynn after they walked past and whispered *"Turn around!"*

"Why?" she whispered back.

"I'm not missing the chance to ride in a tiny elevator with Mick Jagger!" I replied. I had been a Rolling Stones fan since the 1960s and now had an opportunity to literally rub shoulders with the Stones's legendary front man. Lynn was a good sport and turned around with me, and we sauntered casually over to the elevator to wait next to Mick and his companion.

When the elevator arrived, we crammed inside and I was pressed shoulder to shoulder with Mick. Naturally, I tried to act cool, like I didn't even know who he was. From the conversation he was having with his date, it was evident that they had forgotten their car keys in the room and were heading back up to retrieve them. I pushed the button for our floor and it turned out they were going to the same floor. When the elevator reached our floor and the doors opened, they went one way and we went the other, and as soon as they went around a corner, Lynn and I turned around and jumped right back on the elevator, and immediately began laughing like teenagers.

The other European prize I won in this era was the BBVA Foundation Frontiers of Knowledge Award, which is an award given annually by the financial group BBVA in conjunction with the Spanish National Research Council. To receive this prize, I flew with Lynn to Madrid in 2010. We were joined by my daughter Mara, an avid world traveler who is fluent in Spanish. I asked Mara to teach me a few Spanish phrases, so that I could blend in as a local. The only phrase I could consistently remember was *"Dónde está el baño?,"* which is Spanish for *"Where is the bathroom?"* I was determined to use this phrase at some point in the trip.

When we went to the Prado, the legendary museum in the heart of Madrid, I sensed an opportunity and approached one of the information desks, asking *"Dónde está el baño?"* My accent must have been very convincing, because the attendant gave me a long, rambling answer in Spanish. I was too embarrassed to say, *"Oh, I don't actually speak Spanish, I was just trying to show off the one phrase I know,"* so I just nodded and went on my way. I walked a distance, found another information desk and asked again about the bathroom, this time in English.

To facilitate my efforts at blending in with the locals, I also bought a few new pieces of clothing. Spanish men often dress in bold colors, so one of the new pieces I bought for this trip was a bright yellow shirt with a lot of flair. I've got to be honest: I thought I looked damn good in this shirt and was excited to wear it as we went out for dinner our first night in Madrid. While I was getting dressed, the song "I Love My Shirt" by Donovan kept playing in a loop in my head.

As I exited the hotel with Lynn and Mara, I noted a massive flock of pigeons that had assembled on a ledge along the hotel. Shortly after we made it to the street, the pigeons lifted off en masse and headed directly at us, flying in formation like a squadron of World War II bombers coming in for a strafing run. As the pigeons zoomed at our heads, we took evasive action and scattered. I felt my body being pelted with payload after payload as the pigeons screamed past. When the dust settled and the flock was gone, I looked myself over and found that I was covered head to toe in thick, gelatinous pigeon droppings. Amazingly, neither Lynn nor Mara had a drop on them. It was like the pigeons had targeted me in particular. My bold yellow shirt was especially saturated with pigeon droppings, so I assumed that something about my shirt had set the pigeons off. *So much for blending in with the boldly dressed men of Madrid*, I thought to myself as I returned to our hotel room for a quick shower and change of clothes.

The worst part of the pigeon incident was not the soiling of my shirt, but rather the lack of respect shown to me by the pigeons. I had been invited to their country to receive a prestigious award, and instead of treating me with dignity and honor, they had just crapped all over me. It reminded me of another time I was disrespected by the locals years earlier when I was invited to give a keynote lecture at a conference in Rome, Italy. The day after my lecture, I went sightseeing with Lynn on a crowded street in the heart of the city. All of a sudden, I felt a commotion to my right. Lynn was grabbing a teenage boy by the wrist and ripping something out of his hand. The kid wrestled free of Lynn's grip and ran off.

"What the hell was that all about?" I asked.

"You didn't see what happened?" Lynn replied. "That kid pickpocketed you. He reached right inside your blazer and pulled out our passports and plane tickets. I got back the passports and one ticket, but he got away with the other ticket."

This was in the days before electronic ticketing, when it was still important to have a paper ticket, so we needed to get the ticket back somehow. Lynn and I were debating whether we should go to the police, but then we saw the kid who had pickpocketed me standing in the street about a block away with several of his friends. He held up the ticket and brandished it for us to see. I walked within shouting range, and despite his broken English it was clear that he wanted to sell the ticket back to me. A brief negotiation ensued, and I ended up getting the ticket back for the equivalent of fifteen dollars. A number of people on the street just watched this whole scenario play out but did nothing; it was as if getting robbed and extorted was just part of the normal Rome experience.

During other travels in this era, I experienced problems caused not by too little respect from the locals, but rather too much. For instance, I was invited to Tokyo to give a named lecture at one of the universities there, and my hosts prepared a detailed itinerary covering every single minute of my visit. For an entire week, Lynn and I were shepherded everywhere and didn't have a moment to ourselves. Sometimes when you're traveling, you just want a little down time to relax, but on this trip we had chaperones in our presence every second of every day.

On our final day in Tokyo, a young assistant professor accompanied us to the train station. It was our understanding that we would be going to Kyoto to do a little sightseeing on our own before flying home. We tried to say goodbye to our escort outside the train station, but he made clear, in halting English, that he'd been specifically assigned to stay with us for the next few hours to make sure we got on the right train and made the right connection. We then told him directly, in no uncertain terms, that we thanked him for his assistance but would prefer some time on our own. Again, he insisted that his directive was to accompany us to the train. By that time, we were exhausted from spending time with our solicitous hosts and desperately wanted some alone time. Thus, while our escort had his back turned and was talking to the driver of the car, I whispered something in Lynn's ear.

"Don't ask questions, just follow me."

With that, I grabbed my suitcase and took off at a near-run into the train station. Lynn followed behind me. Once inside, we saw an escalator heading down, so we jumped onto it and then took a hard right followed by a hard left followed by another down escalator. I figured we must have lost our escort, but when I turned around and looked back I saw him hustling down the first escalator, chasing after us.

For the next ten minutes, we were on the run. Lynn and I sprinted through the train station, zigzagging at random times, trying to disappear into the crowd and then doubling back to throw our pursuer off our trail. Finally, we hid out in a busy gift shop and watched our escort walk by us, quizzically searching all around the platform. Finally, he gave up and headed back out of the train station.

I have to confess I felt guilty ditching our escort, who seemed like a very nice young man. However, after nearly a week of constantly having people hovering around us, Lynn and I just needed some time to ourselves. It turns out that it *is* possible to be treated with too much respect.

◆

Of all the international cities to which I've traveled during my career at Duke, I've made the most visits to Stockholm, at least a dozen in total. Frequent visits to Stockholm are not uncommon for well-known scientists, as members of the various Nobel committees enjoy inviting potential Nobelists to town in order to meet them in person and see if they have the right stuff. Needless to say, invitations to give scientific talks in Stockholm are *rarely* declined.

My first visit to Stockholm came in 1976 when I was invited to give a lecture at the Karolinska Institute and have dinner with the great Ulf von Euler, a legendary Swedish scientist who many years earlier had discovered noradrenaline (norepinephrine). A decade and a half later, in 1992, I was invited back to the Karolinska to give the Ulf von Euler lecture, which had been named for von Euler after he passed in 1983. I felt honored to give the lecture that was posthumously named for this legend whom I had enjoyed meeting in my earlier visit. I was hosted at the Karolinska by a prominent physiologist who had photos in his office of all the previous scientists who had been invited to give the Ulf von Euler lecture. I noted that more than half of these lecturers had gone on to win the Nobel Prize. My host gave me a brief tour of the photos.

"This guy here, as you know, won the Nobel Prize five years ago. This fellow here won the Prize last year. And this guy here," he said, pointing to my own photo on the wall, "This Lefkowitz guy, we'll just have to wait and see . . ." His voice trailed off and I smiled a taut smile. In case it wasn't already obvious that I was being checked out by the Nobel committee, that fact now seemed to have been made explicit.

In 1996, I was invited back to Stockholm for a Nobel Symposium. All speakers were given thirty minutes, and I gave my normal research seminar focused on the studies my lab was conducting at that time. However, two of the other speakers, Eric Kandel and Paul Greengard, gave very different types of talks. Both gave sweeping talks about their entire careers, grandly framing their work as central to the history of their fields. As it turned out, Kandel and Greengard would share a Nobel Prize (along with Arvid Carlsson) a few years later, so I learned a lesson: the Nobel Symposia were not just regular meetings to talk about your research, but instead were testing grounds in which arguments could be made about why one's body of work might be Nobel-worthy.

Between 2000 and 2012, I was invited back to Stockholm ten times, including several times for Nobel Symposia. After many of these talks, I received highly encouraging feedback from various Nobel Committee members. Each time this happened, I naturally wondered if that might be the year I would finally win a Nobel Prize. Year after year, though, the Nobel announcements came and went without my receiving a call from Stockholm. In October of 2004, Linda Buck and Richard Axel were announced as the winners of the Nobel Prize in Physiology or Medicine for their work identifying the large family of receptors mediating the sense of smell. Their strategy for identifying those receptors was inspired by my lab's work in identifying the adrenergic receptors, and in fact our published sequences for the beta-2 adrenergic and several other receptors had served as the Rosetta Stone for uncovering the olfactory receptors, just as they had for uncovering so many other types of receptors. After Buck and Axel won the Prize, I figured that this was probably the end of the line for my own Nobel hopes: once people start winning Nobel Prizes for studies based on your work, you can't help but feel that you've just been passed over.

With the Shaw Prize, the French prize, the Spanish prize, and others, I had won plenty of prizes in my life. One more award wouldn't make or break my career. Moreover, no true scientist is motivated by the prospect of winning awards. Scientists are motivated by curiosity about how nature works. As the twenty-first century progressed, I felt my own scientific curiosity still burning as intensely as ever. Unlike some scientists I knew who spent almost all their time travelling the globe, my international adventures represented only a small fraction of my time, even though they yielded plenty of good stories. The majority of my days were spent in my lab at Duke, talking with my students and postdocs, and moving my lab's research in interesting new directions. Some of the stories I was most excited about involved studies on beta-arrestins as signaling molecules, and additionally we pursued intensive collaborative efforts to determine the three-dimensional structure of receptors.

TWENTY

The Death Project

The phone rang in my office, and when I answered it I received shocking news: my collaborator, the legendary Harvard structural biologist Don Wiley, was missing. Don and I had been collaborating on trying to determine the three-dimensional structure of the beta-2 adrenergic receptor. In the 1970s, my lab had pioneered the purification of the receptor, and in the 1980s we had discovered the receptor's gene sequence. Now, in the early 2000s, we were collaborating with Wiley's group to perform X-ray crystallography on purified beta-2 receptors in order to see the receptor's structure and understand precisely how molecules like adrenaline bound to it. My lab was adept at purifying receptors and Don Wiley was one of the best X-ray crystallographers in the world, so I felt confident about our chances for success. There was only one problem: Wiley had now vanished without a trace.

Don was an amazing scientist and brilliant wit who lit up every room he entered. He could give a talk about a seemingly dry topic, like the structure of a protein, and weave a spellbinding narrative that would have an audience hanging on his every word. As a storyteller myself, I recognized Don as a kindred spirit and was thrilled to have him as a collaborator. My affection and admiration for Don made his unexplained absence all the more difficult to accept.

Wiley's disappearance became a national news story, so between reading the news and talking with colleagues who knew Don, I became aware of all the details of the case. Don had been at a meeting in Memphis at St. Jude Children's Research Hospital, where he served on a research advisory board. He'd had dinner with some colleagues, and everyone at his table said Don was his usual upbeat and jovial self. Don left the dinner in a rental car to visit his father, who lived in the area, but then never showed up at his father's house. Police found Don's car parked on the Hernando de Soto Bridge, a huge overpass spanning the Mississippi River. One obvious possibility was that Don might have stopped on the bridge and jumped to his death. However, Don had never shown the slightest hint of depression and by all accounts was in especially good spirits that evening.

As weeks passed without any break in the case, conspiracy theories began to pop up. Don was one of the world's top experts on the structure of dangerous viruses, such as the Ebola virus, which led some people to speculate that he may have been kidnapped by terrorists who wanted to develop a biological weapon. This was shortly after the terrorist events of 9/11, so terrorism was very much on everyone's mind. Others speculated that maybe Don knew too much about some sort of dark secret and was murdered. Several other virus experts had died under mysterious circumstances around the same time, which only fueled speculation about Don's case.

About a month after Don's disappearance, his body was found in the Mississippi River about three hundred miles south of Memphis. FBI agents and local law enforcement officials examined his body and also performed a careful examination of his car, which had some damage on the right front end. The official theory of Don's death, put forward by the Shelby County Medical Examiner, was that his car had grazed a post on the bridge, which led him to stop his car and get out to inspect the damage. Somehow, he had then accidentally fallen off the bridge to his death. A large truck may have gone past, creating a strong surge of wind that knocked Don off the bridge. Alternatively, as Don did have an epileptic condition and was prone to the occasional seizure, he may have experienced a seizure event (perhaps related to the stress of hitting the post) and fallen over the railing. In whatever way Don's death actually happened, it was a jolt to the scientific community to lose a man who many thought might win a Nobel Prize in the next few years, and it was especially shocking to me, as we were actively collaborating with his lab.

One of the most macabre aspects of Don's death was that he was actually our third collaborator on the X-ray crystallography project to die unexpectedly. Prior to collaborating with Don on this project, we had been working with Paul Sigler at Yale. Shortly after that collaboration began, the talented postdoctoral fellow who was leading the project, Serge Pares, died tragically (along with his pregnant wife) aboard TWA Flight 800, which exploded and crashed into the Atlantic Ocean shortly after takeoff in 1996. The project continued in the Sigler lab with contributions from several other postdocs. Then, in early 2000, Paul Sigler was walking near the Yale campus one day when he suddenly had a massive heart attack and dropped dead. Paul was a wonderful man and a hell of a scientist, so it was a devastating loss for all who knew him. One of the postdocs in Paul's lab who was working on the project, Ben Spiller, then moved to the lab of Don Wiley at Harvard, and Don expressed an interest in continuing the collaboration with my lab. Thus, when Don's body was pulled out of the Mississippi River on December 20, 2001, he was our third collaborator on this project in six years to have met an untimely demise. In my lab, there was hushed talk about the X-ray crystallography studies being the "Death Project," and concerns were raised that anybody working on this project might be cursed.

Though he had every reason to feel shaken, Ben Spiller was undaunted by talk of a curse. After suffering through the deaths of two consecutive mentors, Ben moved to the lab of yet another famous structural biologist, Stephen Harrison at Harvard, and told me that he wanted to keep working on the project. Amazingly, Steve Harrison was also on board with the idea. Steve had actually taken in quite a few of the mentorless young scientists from Don Wiley's lab and was trying to help them continue their work. I called Steve and offered him the chance to decline this particular project, noting that the last two investigators who took on this collaboration were both now dead. In an act of defiance and bravery, Steve said he didn't believe in curses and was excited about the project, and he insisted on continuing the collaboration with Spiller as the point man.

◆

At the same time as these X-ray crystallography efforts were going on in my lab, we also had a number of other projects that were yielding interesting findings. For example, we were discovering novel cellular proteins that associated with the beta-adrenergic receptors. The distinct sets of binding partners we found for the beta-1 versus beta-2 adrenergic receptors helped to explain certain functional differences between these two receptors that had long been mysterious.[1] Using similar techniques, we discovered a number of cellular binding partners for beta-arrestins. Years earlier, we had found that beta-arrestins could arrest G protein signaling by adrenergic and many other receptors, and subsequently Marc Caron's lab had performed elegant studies demonstrating that beta-arrestins could mediate the removal of receptors from the cell surface in response to overstimulation.[2] In our screens for beta-arrestin binding partners, however, we kept finding proteins that were known to mediate cellular signaling, which didn't make any sense because we were in the mindset that the role of beta-arrestins was to *block* cellular signaling. Around this same time, we also found surprising evidence that beta-arrestin-mediated removal of receptors from the cell surface was important for certain aspects of receptor signaling,[3] which again didn't make sense because the standard model held that removal of receptors from the cell surface should only impair signaling.

Eventually, we had a conceptual breakthrough: we realized that in addition to arresting G protein signaling, beta-arrestins must also initiate a second, distinct wave of signaling coming from the receptors.[4] Given the existence of multiple signaling pathways, it was natural to ask whether it might be possible to differentially activate one pathway over another using distinct receptor ligands. At that time, there was already a small literature about "biased" signaling by G protein–coupled receptors,[5] which is the concept that some drugs are capable of activating certain pathways downstream of a receptor but not others. However, this was mainly discussed in terms of a receptor being able to differentially activate distinct G proteins. I fell in love with the idea that differential activation of signaling by G proteins versus beta-arrestins might be a specific mechanism through which biased signaling occurred.

We explored this idea in studies on both beta-adrenergic and angiotensin receptors, and found that distinct ligands could indeed differentially stimulate signaling mediated by G proteins versus beta-arrestins.[6] To me, these findings about biased ligands were exciting because they suggested the possibility of developing drugs that acted more specifically and had fewer side effects. It now seemed possible to selectively activate just the pathways downstream of a receptor that provided the clinical benefits while avoiding pathways that caused side effects. I was so enamored of these findings that for the first time in my life, I helped to start a company, Trevena, which focused on screening for and developing biased ligands. Three postdoctoral fellows from my lab—Scott DeWire, Jonathan Violin, and Erin Whalen—were the founding scientists of this company. As with many start-up companies, it was a wild ride for Trevena during its first decade, with a lot of ups and downs and growing pains. I no longer have much connection with the company, but Trevena is still actively developing therapeutics and recently had a drug approved by the FDA for clinical use. This drug activates the mu-opioid receptor to decrease severe pain, but, unlike morphine and other traditional mu-opioid activators, this new drug is biased toward G protein signaling and away from beta-arrestin signaling to help reduce side effects. It has been exciting to watch Trevena's efforts to translate the basic research findings about biased signaling into new drugs that will actually help patients.

◆

While my lab's studies on biased signaling were in full swing, we also were purifying large amounts of beta-2 adrenergic receptors on a weekly basis and sending these samples to Ben Spiller in Steve Harrison's lab at Harvard. It was a tough situation for Ben, having lost two mentors in tragic fashion and now doggedly trying to carry on his attempts to solve the crystal structure of the beta-2 receptor. Technically, the project was incredibly demanding, as by definition receptors are squirmy proteins that are prone to rapidly changing conformations. If you think about it, that's what receptors do for a living: rapidly change conformations in response to ligands. Thus, it's incredibly challenging to get a receptor to hold still for a photograph, which is basically what you have to do in order to capture an X-ray crystal structure. After a couple years of work on the project, Ben finally threw in the towel, and my lab moved on completely from the X-ray crystallography efforts because we were so focused on other interesting projects such as the biased signaling work. Thus, when it came to the X-ray crystallography studies, aka the

"Death Project," the bad news was that we were unable to solve the crystal structure of the beta-2 receptor. The good news, though, was that no further deaths were associated with the project: Spiller, Harrison, and the folks in my lab who were pursuing these studies all survived to tell the tale.

A couple of years later, in 2006, Brian Kobilka and I shared a visiting lectureship at the University of Illinois at Urbana-Champaign. This joint lectureship provided Brian and me with some quality time to catch up with each other. Brian had been on the Stanford faculty for about sixteen years at that time and achieved a fair amount of research success, although not the transcendent success that I (and many others) had predicted for him when he left my lab in 1990.

At a dinner together during our visit in Illinois, Brian confided to me that he had been focusing much of his lab's efforts on solving a crystal structure for the beta-2 adrenergic receptor. I told him that we also had pursued efforts in this area for a while but dropped the project several years earlier because of concerns that success might not be possible with the current state of the technology. Brian said he also had encountered many technical difficulties and was simply hoping to get a crystal structure before he retired, perhaps at some point in the next twenty years. When Brian said this, I patted myself on the back for having the wisdom to drop the X-ray crystallography project and focus on other lines of research, because it seemed crazy to labor for twenty years trying to achieve a goal that might end up being just a pipe dream.

About a year later, in the spring of 2007, I received a call from Brian with some surprising news. He said that his lab had achieved a number of technical breakthroughs and now had a crystal structure for the beta-2 adrenergic receptor! However, there was a problem: he was mired in authorship issues with his collaborator Ray Stevens, and they were unable to come to an agreement about the order of authors on the first paper describing the new crystal structure. Over the years, I have received many such phone calls from lab alumni concerning authorship issues, so I listened intently to Brian's specific case.

Author lists on scientific papers are often long, and the greatest prestige is given to the first and last authors. The first author is usually the junior scientist who performed most of the experiments, whereas the last author is traditionally the senior scientist who offered overall direction to the project. When two or more labs collaborate on a large project, there can be conflict over which lab should be rewarded with the first and last author positions on the resultant manuscript. In the case of the beta-2 receptor structure, Brian told me that he was considering dividing up the findings into two back-to-back manuscripts, with his lab having first and last authorship on one paper and Stevens's lab taking the premier authorship positions on the other. I told Brian that I thought this was a bad idea because the work would have greater impact as a single comprehensive report. As it turned out, Brian ignored my advice, wrote the two papers to spread out the authorships, and everything worked out fine. Subsequently, I joked with Brian that this strategy has probably been a major key to the success he's had in his career: he asks for my advice, and then always does the opposite.

In November 2007, Brian and his collaborators published their back-to-back papers in *Science* describing the crystal structure of the beta-2 adrenergic receptor.[7] These papers were a technical tour de force. Brian's lab innovated at every step of the process: improving the purification process to obtain much larger quantities of pure receptor than was previously possible, engineering the receptor to be much more stable than it normally was, and a dozen other technical twists that other scientists couldn't even dream up, much less actually attempt. This breakthrough had an enormous impact on the field, as everyone now saw the path forward to solving the crystal structures for the hundreds of other G protein–coupled receptors encoded in the human genome. I was dazzled by this quantum leap in technical capability and absolutely thrilled for Brian, who had gambled a great deal in pursuing these structural studies and now saw his gamble pay off in the biggest way imaginable. What I didn't know at the time, however, was that an even more dramatic advance was on the way.

In the spring of 2011, I was attending the annual meeting of the National Academy of Sciences, at which the names of the newly elected members were about to be announced. Election to the academy represents one of the highest honors bestowed on American scientists. I had nominated Brian several years earlier and each year I had been advocating for his election. In 2011, Brian finally received enough votes to be elected, and right after the final vote I had the honor and pleasure of calling him to tell him the good news. I stepped outside the National Academy of Sciences headquarters in Washington, D. C., and called Brian on my cell phone. It was 9:00 A.M. in Washington, which meant it was 6:00 A.M. California time. When I called, Brian's wife, Tong Sun, answered his phone.

"Hey Tong Sun, this is Bob Lefkowitz. I'm calling to congratulate Brian on the good news."

"Oh, you heard," Tong Sun replied.

I was dumbfounded, because there was no way that Brian could already know about his election to the National Academy, which had happened just minutes before I called him.

"What are you talking about?" I asked.

"About the structure," Tong Sun answered. Again, I was dumbfounded. This conversation felt like an Abbott and Costello routine.

"What structure?"

"The structure of the receptor with the G protein," said Tong Sun. "They solved it last week. I assumed that's why you want to congratulate him."

"Well, that's wonderful news Tong Sun," I said. "But that is *not* why I'm calling. So please put Brian on."

"He's still sleeping," said Tong Sun.

"Well, wake him up!" I cheerfully bellowed. I knew that Brian wouldn't mind being roused to receive such happy news. Moreover, now that I knew he had solved the structure of the complex between the receptor and G protein, I wanted to talk to him about it.

A few months later, in July 2011, Brian's group published a lead article in *Nature* reporting the crystal structure of the beta-2 adrenergic receptor in complex with a G protein.[8] This work was done collaboratively with several other labs, including the labs of Roger Sunahara, which had provided the purified G proteins used to achieve the docked structure, and Yiorgo Skiniotis, which had performed crucial electron microscopy work. This work was even more of a tour de force than the 2007 papers reporting the first structure of the beta-2 receptor. If you think it's hard getting one squirmy protein to sit still for a photograph, try getting two hyperkinetic proteins to hold still and pose together long enough to take a perfect photo. The technical advances in Brian's 2011 paper were staggering, and the structure was absolutely beautiful. Many new insights into how receptors work could be gleaned from this structure, and Brian went on a barnstorming tour to describe his lab's latest findings.

That summer, I was speaking at a Nobel Symposium in Stockholm. It was my tenth visit to Stockholm in eleven years. Brian was not giving a talk at the meeting, but people were talking about him. He had just shown his receptor-G protein structure at a European biophysics meeting, and Gunnar von Heijne, a member of the Nobel Committee for Chemistry, had witnessed the presentation. He then returned to Stockholm for the Nobel Symposium where I was speaking, and when I chatted with him during a break in the meeting I could tell that he was over the moon about Brian's latest breakthrough. The sentiment seemed to be shared by several other members of the Nobel Chemistry Committee who were attending the meeting. Of course, I had long ago given up trying to read into comments made by Nobel Committee members, as I had received many enthusiastic comments over the years from various Nobel Committee members without ever being tapped for a Nobel Prize.

That October, the Nobel Prize announcements came and went, and neither Brian nor I received a call from Stockholm. As usual, numerous people asked me questions about whether I would ever win. I kept thinking about what Al Gilman said after he won his Nobel: *"The best thing about winning the Nobel Prize is never again having to answer the question, 'When are you going to win the Nobel Prize?'"* Admittedly, my situation in 2011 was not as bad as it had been in 2003, when my local paper, the *Durham Herald-Sun*, had run a front-page, above-the-fold photograph of me with a headline that read, NOBEL CALLING? ALAS, NOT THIS YEAR. At the time, I was thinking: *who else in the world makes headlines for NOT winning the Nobel Prize?* In 2003, that headline had bothered me a little bit. By 2011, I was just enjoying my day-to-day work as a scientist and mentor, and was absolutely done with worrying about awards.

TWENTY-ONE

Eat More Chocolate, Win More Nobel Prizes

I was awakened by an elbow to my ribs. The clock read 5:00 A.M. and the room was dark. I pulled the earplugs out of my ears and glanced over at Lynn, who had just elbowed me awake and was holding the phone toward me. Usually, when you get awakened by a call this early in the morning, it's bad news. This time, it was just the opposite.

"Stockholm is calling," Lynn intoned. I took the phone from Lynn as I rubbed the sleep out of my eyes.

"Hello?"

"Professor Lefkowitz?" said a woman with a Swedish accent. "I'm going to put Professor Staffan Normark on the line. He's the permanent secretary of the Swedish Academy of Sciences, and he has some good news for you."

"Okay, thank you," I said as my mind raced. The date was Wednesday, October 10, 2012. I had always thought that if I ever won the Nobel Prize, I would win it in Physiology or Medicine. However, the Physiology or Medicine Prize for 2012 had been announced two days earlier, and it had gone to Shinya Yamanaka and John Gurdon for their work on reprogramming mature cells into stem cells. When that prize had been announced, I figured it had ended any possibility of my winning a Nobel for another year. Now, though, I was getting a call from the Swedish Academy of Sciences, which was completely unexpected.

"Good morning Professor Lefkowitz!" exclaimed Staffan Normark as he came on the line. He congratulated me and stated that I would be receiving the Nobel Prize in Chemistry. I thanked him and asked *"Can you tell me if I'll be sharing the prize with anyone?"*

"Yes, you'll be sharing the prize with Brian Kobilka," Normark replied.

"That's wonderful," I said. I could hardly imagine anything better than sharing a Nobel Prize with one of my trainees. "Can I call Brian?"

"No," said Normark quickly. "We called you first, so please wait at least fifteen minutes for us to call Professor Kobilka to give him the news. And other than calling Professor Kobilka, we ask that you please don't call anyone else for the next hour. We'll be having a press conference to announce the news at approximately 6:00 A.M. Eastern Standard Time, so please don't call any friends or relatives until that time."

I promised that I would remain incommunicado. Normark handed me off to talk with Sven Lidin, the chair of the Nobel Committee for Chemistry, followed by several other members of the Committee who wanted to offer their brief congratulations. Then, when I hung up, everything was quiet. It was a surreal feeling, sitting there in bed, having just received this bombshell news but not being able to tell anyone other than Lynn. I wanted to call my kids, I wanted to call other family and friends, but I was not allowed to tell anyone until after the press conference.

"Well, we can't talk to anyone, so I guess I'll just go make some coffee," I said to Lynn as I rolled out of bed and headed to the kitchen.

The one person I was allowed to call was Brian, so after waiting a half hour I phoned Brian and we had a brief conversation. Brian told me that he had initially ignored the call from Stockholm, assuming it was a wrong number or prank call. When the phone kept ringing, he ultimately answered, and still thought it might be a prank until Normark handed the phone around to the various members of the Nobel Committee. Brian realized that it would have to be quite an elaborate gag to assemble five different people with convincing Swedish accents, so after hearing the voices of the various members of the Nobel Committee, Brian was finally convinced of the authenticity of the call.

I was amused by Brian's tale, but also had something serious I wanted to say to him. I felt like I had been on the cusp of winning the Nobel Prize for many years, but in my view Brian's recent crystal structures had represented the critical final step of the journey that had put things over the top.

"I'm pretty sure I wouldn't have won without you," I told Brian.

"I think you've got that backward," replied Brian with characteristic humility.

Shortly after I signed off from talking to Brian, I received a call back from Stockholm that allowed me to participate in the press conference via phone. I answered a few perfunctory questions from journalists about the significance of our research and then signed off. My plan was to immediately start calling my family. Before I could place a single call, though, the phone rang again. I answered and found myself live on the air of a morning radio show in New York City. They had seen in the Nobel announcement that I was a native New Yorker, so they wanted to talk to me about my upbringing in New York in addition to chatting about my research. When I hung up from talking to the morning show, the phone rang again within a few seconds, and it was the *New York Times*.

After that, it was the *Washington Post*, the *Durham Herald-Sun*, and a half-dozen other news outlets in rapid succession.

National Public Radio called, and the morning hosts asked me what I had planned to be doing that day before I received the call from Stockholm.

"Well, I *was* going to get a haircut this morning," I said as the hosts roared with laughter. "If you could see me, you'd see it's quite a necessity. But I'm afraid the haircut will probably have to be postponed. It's okay—my wife told me that 'slightly disheveled' is a good look for a Nobel Prize winner."

In between these calls from the media, Ralph Snyderman somehow snuck a call through to offer brief congratulations. Rick Cerione also snuck through a call in between media outlets. I was still trying to call my kids, but every time I hung up the phone it began buzzing again within a second or two. Finally, I got through to my sons David and Josh to tell them the news. By the time I got through to Noah, he had already seen the news on his Facebook feed and called my daughter Mara in San Francisco to wake her up and tell her.

"Dad won the Nobel!" he shouted in Mara's ear.

"No he didn't," Mara replied, slightly annoyed. "They gave it out on Monday and he didn't win this year." After learning that I had won the Chemistry Prize, rather than the Physiology or Medicine Prize, Mara then called her sister, Cheryl, to tell her, and so three of my five kids had already heard the news before I could get ahold of them that morning.

I drove to work at 9:00 A.M. and was greeted with a surprise before I even parked my car. My parking garage entrance featured a huge, multicolored sign that read CONGRATS BOB! To this day, I have no idea who put that sign there. When I walked into my office, it was already filled with well-wishers: folks from my lab, people from down the hall, and friends from all across campus. It was like a giant party, and the room exploded with applause and cheers when I walked in. Definitely a nice way to start the workday! I went into full schmoozing mode and began to make my way around the balloon-filled room. At 11:00 A.M., I was ushered down the hall for cake and champagne in the conference room. I got some laughs by noting that the cake was obviously a rush job, as "Lefkowitz" was misspelled, and this only added to the merriment.

At 1:00 P.M., I headed across the Duke campus for the official press conference. I made a brief statement and took questions from the media. One journalist noted that I was a native New Yorker and asked if I was a Yankees fan. I said yes and noted I was such a huge fan growing up that I could still recite from memory the uniform numbers and batting order of the Yankees starting lineup from the 1950s. *"Well, go ahead and recite it!"* the journalist said. So I did:

Hank Bauer, right field, #9
Phil Rizzuto, shortstop, #10
Mickey Mantle, center field, #7 (my favorite)
Yogi Berra, catcher, #8
Moose Skowron, first base, #53
Gene Woodling, left field, #14
Gil McDougald, second base, #12
Andy Carey, third base, #6
Whitey Ford, pitcher, #16

Somehow, my ability to recite the Yankees lineup became a national news story. It was mentioned in numerous outlets, especially the New York papers. It had just been a brief off-the-cuff moment at a news conference, but for some reason it became a central part of the Nobel Prize coverage that day.

At 4:00 P.M., there was a reception held at the beautiful Washington Duke Inn just across the road from the Duke campus. An email was sent out during the day inviting all Duke faculty and staff to attend this event, and several hundred people showed up. It was fantastic to have the chance to catch up with so many friends and colleagues from across the campus, and the energy in the room was unbelievable. I was impressed because it was quite a gala event for something thrown together on such short notice. I talked at the reception with someone from the Duke Communications Office, and they told me they were able to act so quickly because they had trained over the years for certain emergency responses. Specifically, my winning the Nobel Prize was one of the emergency scenarios for which they had prepared. It turns out that I was the first Nobel Laureate ever from Duke University, so the whole Duke campus was ready to celebrate if and when I won the prize.

Later in the day, I finally had a chance to check my email and found that I had received more than 700 messages following the Nobel announcement. Ultimately, I would receive more than 1,500 congratulatory emails that week; I worked with my staff in the subsequent weeks to make sure that I replied to each and every email. The very first email in the queue had come exactly at 6:00 A.M. and was from the legendary Swedish neuroscientist Tomas Hökfelt. As a member of the Royal Swedish Academy of Sciences, he had advance warning of the Nobel announcement. His note to me began, *"Dear Bob, I already wrote this message and had it ready to go because I wanted to be the first to congratulate you."* He had waited for the official announcement and then pressed the send button immediately. I also received emails from friends, family, colleagues, neighbors, classmates from all phases of my education (including some I hadn't seen since elementary school), and even random people named Lefkowitz. One touching message I received was from a guy named Gary Lefkowitz in San Francisco. It read:

"Dear Robert—All of us with the surname Lefkowitz are standing a little bit taller today thanks to your remarkable career, your achievements and awards. My parents, Abraham and Fannie, arrived to Ellis Island aboard the USS *Marine Flasher* in 1946. We may be distant relatives or not, but if you ever get to San Francisco, you're family! Our heartfelt congratulations go out to you—Gary."

In addition to all the emails, I received countless phone calls over the next few days. Needless to say, these calls had to be screened by my assistant, Donna Addison, who decided on the calls I would take right away versus the callers who could just leave a message. One call that Donna put through without hesitation was from the legendary Duke basketball coach Mike Krzyzewski. At that stage of his career, Coach K had already won four national championships with Duke and two gold medals coaching Team USA at the Olympics. I had been a Duke basketball season ticket holder since the 1970s, but never had occasion to interact with Krzyzewski. Thus, it was a delight to have the chance to schmooze with him for a half hour on the phone when he called me a couple of days after the Nobel announcement.

Coach K was incredibly gracious during our phone conversation and said that he felt a special kinship with me: he was the first person to bring a basketball national championship to Duke and I was the first person to bring a Nobel Prize to our university. Given this connection, Coach K said, nothing would be more appropriate than for me to be honored at Cameron Indoor Stadium, the storied arena where Duke basketball games are played. As it turned out, there would be a special event the following week, called "Countdown to Craziness," which would mark the official start of basketball season. This event would include player introductions and an intrasquad scrimmage in front of a packed house at Cameron. Coach K suggested that I should be honored in some way at this event.

"What do you have in mind?" I asked him.

"You'll see," he replied cryptically.

Coach K told me to bring a few guests, so I showed up the following week at Countdown to Craziness with Lynn as well as a couple of members of my lab, Seungkirl Ahn and Jeff Kovacs, who were both die-hard

Duke basketball fans. Kovacs was such an insane fan that when he was a graduate student he was known as "Mullet Man" because he attended every Duke home game decked out in Duke gear and wearing a huge wig that was shaped like an over-the-top mullet. It was a thrill for all of us to sit behind the Duke bench and chat with Coach K before the proceedings began.

The lights went down and the player introductions began. Each player came out dancing to a high-energy song after his name was called, with all 10,000 fans going crazy. I was getting a little nervous because I had not prepared any dance moves for the occasion and was wondering if the crowd would be disappointed if I didn't shimmy my way out on the court when I was introduced. When the player introductions finished, the lights came up and Coach K walked to center court with a microphone.

"Now I want to bring out a special guest. I'm sure you all saw on the news last week that Dr. Robert Lefkowitz became the first Nobel Laureate in the history of Duke University. I'd like to invite Dr. Lefkowitz to join us on the court."

With that, I climbed over the railing and walked out onto the court as the crowd went berserk. I received handshakes and high-fives from all the Duke players, feeling the shortest I have ever felt in my life as I walked amongst this pack of giants. Coach K then took out a #1 Duke jersey that said LEFKOWITZ on the back (spelled correctly!), and the players helped me to put on the jersey as the crowd roared appreciatively. Coach K and the players then began to walk off the court and I followed them, but Coach K waved me back to center court to soak in the cheers for bit longer.

The students who attend Duke basketball games are known as "Cameron Crazies," and they are renowned for their loud chants during the games. As I stood at center court reveling in the thunderous applause, I heard the students chanting something and pointing at me, but I couldn't quite make out what they were saying. Finally, I realized that they were rhythmically chanting, *"He's so smart! He's so smart! He's so smart!"* I cracked up and raised my arms in the air, which led the students to roar even louder.

After basking in the ovation for a few more seconds, I headed off the court and took my seat next to Lynn and the others right behind the Duke bench. The intrasquad scrimmage began and we were treated throughout the entire game to a running commentary by Coach K. *"Watch this move, he's been working on it the whole offseason,"* Coach K would say. *"By the way, we're recruiting this guy's cousin, but I don't think we're going to get him."* As a Duke basketball fan, it was a delight to hear all this inside information about the team and also be privy to insight after insight from one of the greatest basketball minds in history.

It was a magical evening to cap off an unbelievable week. I had been at Duke for nearly forty years at that point, and many different people in the Duke community had contributed to the success of my research program over the years. It felt wonderful to be sharing the Nobel Prize with everyone at Duke and to feel the buzz and excitement that had been generated all over the Duke campus by the news of this award. It was like a dream come true.

◆

On October 10, 2012, the very day on which I received the call from Stockholm, an article was published in the prestigious *New England Journal of Medicine* entitled "Chocolate Consumption, Cognitive Function, and Nobel Laureates."[1] This piece, written by Franz Messerli, M.D., from Columbia University, reported a surprisingly robust correlation between chocolate consumption per capita in various countries and the number of Nobel Prizes per capita won by those countries. People in Switzerland, for instance, eat a huge amount of chocolate per person and also win a large number of Nobel Prizes for such a small country. In contrast, chocolate consumption in China is very low and China has few Nobel Laureates despite a very large population. The USA is in the middle, with average chocolate consumption as well as an average number of Nobel Laureates per capita.

This article about the connection between chocolate consumption and Nobel Prizes caught my attention because in 2012, the year I won the prize, I had greatly increased my own chocolate consumption. I have always loved dark chocolate. However, given my genetic predisposition toward cardiac disease, I have been highly disciplined about my diet for most of my adult life and avoided sweets. For many years, I would buy bars of dark chocolate but only allow myself to enjoy a single square from these bars a couple of evenings per week. I was a model of chocolate-eating self-restraint, going through an average of one chocolate bar every couple of weeks.

In the summer of 2012, I had a physical where everything looked great. My weight was perfect. My cholesterol numbers were sensational. My surgically repaired heart was performing well. This glowing physical report prompted me to make a radical announcement to Lynn.

"I've been thinking about it and come to the decision that I'm now going to eat a square of dark chocolate *every* evening rather than just twice a week," I said to Lynn. My rationale was: *what the hell, I'm sixty-nine years old and my numbers all look fine. Why not live a little?*

"You are totally out of control!" Lynn replied in feigned alarm.

I began enjoying my dark chocolate on a nightly basis in July 2012. Three months later, I won the Nobel Prize. Coincidence? I think not. This episode is yet another data point for researchers like Dr. Messerli to consider in their analyses of the close connection between chocolate consumption and Nobel Prizes. In fact, my experience illustrates two important points about this phenomenon:

> i) *The effect of chocolate is dose-dependent.* I've eaten chocolate my entire life, but it wasn't until I increased my weekly dose that the Nobel-Prize-inducing effect kicked in.

ii) The effect of chocolate is rapidly acting. Once I increased my dose, I won the Nobel Prize within several months. This suggests that even a brief elevation in dose is sufficient to gain the full benefits.

Having finally received my chocolate-provoked call from Stockholm, I realized that I now had a lot to do. The Nobel Prizes are announced in early October each year, but the actual ceremony takes place on the anniversary of Alfred Nobel's death, December 10. This allows two months for each new Nobel Laureate to prepare for their upcoming visit to Stockholm, and let me tell you, there are a lot of things that need to be prepared.

Without a doubt, the two months between the call from Stockholm and the Nobel ceremony were the busiest two months of my life. First of all, each new Laureate is required to write a detailed biography for the Nobel website. I didn't happen to have a detailed biography laying around at the time, so it took quite a bit of time and effort to craft that document. Secondly, all Laureates are required to film videos for the Nobel website in which they discuss their prizewinning work, and a lot of hours go into preparing for the filming of these videos. Thirdly, all Laureates are required to give a public Nobel Lecture about their prize-winning endeavors in the days just before the Nobel ceremony. These lectures are recorded and posted on the Nobel website for future generations to watch, so needless to say it's important to practice one's speech assiduously in order to make sure it's worthy of the occasion.

Beyond the intensive efforts required to put together the biography, video, and lecture, there are also a host of other demands on the time of every newly minted Laureate. Travel arrangements must be made, new clothes must be purchased, and congratulatory messages must be answered. Moreover, decisions need to be made about the allocation of tickets to the various Nobel events. For example, each Laureate is allowed to bring their spouse to the Nobel Banquet and also invite fourteen additional guests. In my case, I decided that my five children had to attend, along with their partners, which accounted for ten tickets. This meant that out of dozens of close family members, friends, and colleagues whom I knew would love to attend the Nobel Banquet, I could only invite four of them. With an endless string of difficult decisions of this type to be made, my anxiety levels were through the roof. The best analogy I could offer for the stress of preparing to receive a Nobel Prize would be the stress of planning a large wedding: it's a happy occasion, to be sure, but still very stressful because there are so many details to obsess over and so many things that can go awry.

Before I knew it, the calendar had turned to December and it was time to go. The trip that followed was a whirlwind unlike anything I have experienced in my life.

TWENTY-TWO

Nobel Week

B rian Kobilka was looking sharp. We were cooling our heels
outside the Oval Office in the White House, waiting to meet
with President Obama, and I was admiring Brian's perfectly
tailored new suit. He was usually a pretty casual dresser, so I commented
on his stylish new duds. Brian smiled sheepishly and made a confession.

"After we got the call from Stockholm, Tong Sun hired two personal
shoppers. One for her and one for me."

I expressed my admiration at Tong Sun's managerial skills. When she
worked in my lab, she was always meticulously organized as a scientist, and
apparently her organizational prowess also extended to travel preparations.
Hiring personal shoppers to get ready for this trip was an act of pure genius;
why didn't I think of that? Lynn had been pulling out her hair trying to
squeeze in shopping trips amongst the hundreds of other things we had
to get done, so it would've been money well spent for her to have had some
help from a personal shopper for a few weeks.

The doors to the Oval Office opened up and we were ushered inside. It was a longstanding tradition for American Nobelists to meet with the president before heading to Stockholm, and this year there was an especially large crop of Laureates from the USA. Five of us filed into the Oval Office with our spouses: in addition to Brian and me, there was David Wineland, who shared the prize in Physics, and Alvin Roth and Lloyd Shapley, who shared the prize in Economics. President Obama, a Nobel Laureate himself from several years earlier, greeted us warmly, and we chatted for twenty minutes or so. It was very satisfying to have some time with Obama, a president I greatly admired, since I didn't get to meet him during my last White House visit. When it was time to leave, we moved toward the door and I was the last to exit the Oval Office. I grabbed Obama's arm as we shook hands.

"I gotta tell you, Mr. President, I'm a huge fan of your wife Michelle."

"Hey, get in line!" joked Obama with a huge smile, referencing recent media reports about his wife's approval rating being higher than his own. Just as this exchange occurred, Pete Souza, the official photographer of the Obama White House, snapped a shot of the two of us warmly shaking hands and smiling broadly. The photo became a favorite of mine and later would hang in my office.

Shortly after the White House visit, we were on a plane to Stockholm. We landed in the middle of a howling snowstorm, and from the moment the plane touched down it was like we were in a fairy tale. The captain said over the loudspeaker, *"Ladies and gentleman, it is my pleasure to tell you that we have one of this year's Nobel Laureates, Dr. Robert Lefkowitz, and his wife on the flight."* The entire plane burst into applause and I gave a little wave. The guy sitting across the aisle from me did a double take, staring at me like he'd seen a ghost. The captain continued, *"Out of respect for Dr. and Mrs. Lefkowitz, I would be greatly appreciative if you could please allow them to deplane first."*

Lynn and I felt self-conscious, but took our bags and headed down the aisle. We were greeted at the cabin door by dignitaries from the Royal Swedish Academy and then exited the plane down a flight of stairs directly onto the snow-covered tarmac, where our Nobel limousine was waiting. This limo was a custom twin-turbo BMW 750 with the Nobel insignia on the outside and every imaginable luxury on the inside: full wet bar, flat-screen television, and lavishly comfortable seats. Our driver said that he would be our personal chauffeur, and this car would be our ride for the entirety of Nobel Week.

We drove to the edge of the airport grounds to something called the "VIP terminal." It was like a posh club at the airport reserved for the welcoming of foreign dignitaries and heads of state. Lynn and I walked into the opulent room, and nobody else was there except for a fleet of attendants who offered us hors d'oeuvres and drinks. We were soon joined by several members of the Nobel Committee and Royal Swedish Academy, and after schmoozing for a bit we were notified that we had been magically cleared through customs and our luggage had somehow been retrieved, so we could now head to our hotel.

We drove in our Nobel limo to the legendary Grand Hotel, which has hosted the Nobel Laureates since the prizes began being awarded in 1901. As soon as I stepped out of the limo at the entrance of the Grand Hotel, I was swarmed by paparazzi. Flashbulbs were popping and people were thrusting notebooks at me trying to get autographs. I was stunned by the chaotic scene. Scientists are not used to being treated like rock stars, but during Nobel Week in Stockholm, Laureates receive the full rock star treatment. I signed a few autographs, posed for a few photos, and then headed into the Grand Hotel to escape the madness.

The most striking thing about Nobel Week is how smoothly everything runs. The Swedes have been giving out Nobel Prizes for more than 110 years, so by now the whole operation runs like clockwork. On the first day, for instance, all the male Laureates had to get fitted for white-tie tuxedos. These ultra-formal tuxedos differ from the regular black-tie variety in having all sorts of extra layers, buttons, and other sartorial add-ons. Laureates are required to wear a specific type of white-tie tuxedo provided by the Nobel Foundation, such that all men in the ceremony are dressed in identical splendor. During my fitting at a special tailoring shop, I was attended to by an entire squadron of tailors who ran a precision drill in taking my measurements and tweaking my tuxedo to perfection.

We were given an itinerary for the week in which every single hour of every single day was laid out for us in excruciating detail. For each block of time, we were told where to be, what to wear, and who should accompany us. The entries on the extensive itinerary all looked like this:

> Thursday, December 6th
> 9:40–11:45 A.M.
> *Laureates get together at Nobel Museum*
> Guests: Laureate, Spouse, Close Family, Attendant
> Dress Code: Business Suit/Dress or Two-Piece Suit for Laureate
> All Others: Casual

During our visit to the Nobel Museum, we engaged in one of the most eccentric traditions associated with the Nobel Prizes: chair signing. We were told that it was a longstanding custom for all Laureates to go to the museum café and sign the underside of one of the café chairs. Thus, if you ever find yourself in Stockholm getting a cup of coffee at the Nobel Museum, you should look at the undersides of the chairs to make sure you pick a good Laureate to sit on.

Everywhere I went in Stockholm, I was instantly recognized. Random people whipped out their smartphones and asked for selfies. A pack of high school students at the Nobel Museum freaked out when they saw me and began shrieking as if seeing Mick Jagger backstage at a Stones concert in the 1970s. I'll be honest: this instant celebrity status was disorienting. It also made it challenging to get in and out of the Grand Hotel due to the density of paparazzi and fans who were camped out at the hotel's entrances. It was rough on Brian and me, but even worse for Shinya Yamanaka because of the insane level of attention he received from the Japanese paparazzi, the most intense and numerous of all journalists in attendance. In fact, Brian and I came to realize that the best time to leave the Grand Hotel was right after Yamanaka, because he would attract such a massive media scrum that it made it possible for others to sneak past without drawing much notice.

On Friday, December 7, I had to sit for a long, recorded interview in the afternoon, and then in the evening there was a dinner hosted by the Royal Swedish Academy. I sat next to one of the members of the Nobel Committee for Chemistry, and we discussed why I had won the Prize in Chemistry. He joked, *"There was a tug of war between us and the Committee for Physiology or Medicine as to who would have the honor of giving you the prize . . . and we won!"*

The reality is that the research for which Brian and I were sharing the prize could best be described as biochemistry, the study of the chemistry of living things. However, there is no Nobel Prize in biochemistry. In the twenty-first century, almost half of Nobel Prizes in Chemistry so far have been given to biochemists who, like Brian and me, skew more toward biology than chemistry. This fact drives many pure chemists crazy, as they argue that the Nobel Prize in Chemistry should go to people who are authentic chemists. The counterargument, though, is that much of the most exciting research in the world these days is being done at the interface between biology and chemistry. Thus, it's not surprising that there has been a blurring of the lines in recent years between the traditional domains of biology and chemistry in major awards such as the Nobel Prizes.

As the Royal Swedish Academy dinner wound down, I had a few minutes to chat with Brian. Our Nobel Lectures were the next morning, so I asked Brian if he was planning to go to bed early. *"No, actually it's going to be a late night for me,"* he replied. *"I'm still working on my slides."* I stared at Brian in disbelief. We were just about to give the biggest talks of our lives, which would be recorded and viewed for many years by future generations, and he was going to pull an all-nighter the night before to finalize his presentation? In contrast, I had practiced my talk dozens of times and honed it to such perfection that I could consistently deliver it in exactly thirty minutes (the requested length) plus or minus ten seconds. Apparently, though, Brian was still making last-minute changes.

The next morning, I was feeling loose before my lecture. The only nervousness I felt was for Brian. As an introvert, he was not a natural public speaker in any case, and now he was sleep-deprived because he had just stayed up much of the night working on his slides. He seemed tight as we took the stage at Aula Magna, the magnificent all-wood auditorium on the campus of Stockholm University. A standing-room-only audience of 1,500 people was waiting expectantly, and more than a dozen cameras were trained on the stage to capture every word we said and every gesture we made.

My lecture was first, and I ran through all my greatest hits. The crowd exploded with applause as I finished and I bounded off the stage on a high. Throughout my talk, I enjoyed seeing dozens of familiar faces in the crowd, as a large contingent of my former trainees had made the trek to Stockholm to enjoy the Nobel festivities. Many of my trainees were sitting right up front, and I had been chatting with them just before my lecture, so it felt almost like I was giving a lab meeting presentation, albeit with a thousand extra guests sitting in.

Now it was Brian's turn. He started tentatively and, like any mentor watching a protégé make an important presentation, I was feeling anxious on his behalf. As Brian's talk went on, though, he began to warm up. His breakthrough crystal structure of the beta-2 adrenergic receptor had required special antibodies made by llamas,[1] so Brian showed a cute photo of him posing next to the llama that had produced the critical antibodies. The llama photo got a huge laugh. Brian also showed a selfie he took with Roger Sunahara and his other collaborators immediately after they first saw the crystal structure of the beta-2 receptor in complex with its G protein. Everyone in the snapshot is smiling ear-to-ear like a team that just won a championship, and this photo also got laughs from the audience. Overall, Brian's talk was wonderful and I could not have been more proud of him. I was thinking about what a long way he had come as a public speaker from that first national meeting in the late 1980s where he had fought off a panic attack during his talk and left the stage drenched in sweat.

The evening after my Nobel Lecture was the only evening free on my schedule, so I had arranged to have dinner with all of my family members who had come to Stockholm: Lynn, my five kids, their partners, two of my grandchildren, my cousins Ellen and Judy, and a few other family members and friends who had made the trip. This dinner was held at the Grand Hotel in a spectacular room with floor-to-ceiling windows that afforded breathtaking views of the Baltic Sea. A light snow was falling and the ambience was straight out of a fairy tale. Just after dinner, my daughter Mara's boyfriend, Eric, came up to me and asked if we could talk outside on the balcony. As we stepped outside into the frigid night air, Eric seemed uncharacteristically nervous. Finally he spoke.

"I am planning to ask for Mara's hand in marriage, but first I wanted to get your blessing," he said. A smile immediately broke over my face, as I was pleased to hear this news for three reasons: first, I really liked Eric; second, they had already been together for five years; and finally, none of us were getting any younger. I put my hand on Eric's shoulder and replied enthusiastically.

"Well, I didn't know that people asked for blessings anymore. But I've always had the highest regard for you, Eric, and honestly I'd be thrilled if you and Mara got married."

Eric thanked me and then said he planned to go diamond shopping the next day. He thought this Stockholm trip was a magical experience and he wanted to purchase a diamond in Stockholm to offer to Mara as an engagement ring. Eric also promised that he would propose to Mara in a low-key manner.

"I know that this is your week, Bob, and the focus should be on you," Eric said. "So I promise I'll find a private, quiet moment to make my proposal."

The next day—Saturday, December 9—was a highlight of the trip because Brian and I organized a lunchtime reception for all of our trainees and collaborators who had made the trip to Stockholm. We gathered in an ornate room in the Grand Hotel, and Brian and I held court for several hours. It was such a pleasure to see so many familiar faces and have the chance to joke around with so many old friends during this special occasion. In my view, I was receiving the Nobel Prize on behalf of all the members of my lab over the years: they were the ones who actually did the experiments and in many cases had key ideas that led to our breakthrough discoveries. Thus, nothing could be more appropriate than to share some extended time together with my colleagues the day before I actually received the prize.

Finally, the big day arrived: Sunday, December 10, the day of the Nobel Ceremony and Nobel Banquet.[2] In the morning, Lynn and I climbed into our Nobel limo and drove in a procession of other limos to the Stockholm Concert Hall for the Nobel Ceremony rehearsal. This event was like a wedding rehearsal, except much bigger and more complicated. Everyone had to practice lining up and marching into the hall in precise formation. We were instructed to take our seats onstage, in the front row straight across from where the royal family would be seated. After our citation was read by a member of the appropriate prize committee, we were instructed to walk across the stage and bow three times: once to the king, once to the dignitaries onstage, and once to the audience. This event was such a full rehearsal that they even had actors playing the different members of the royal family, including a guy playing the king who actually sort of looked like the king.

After the rehearsal, we headed back to the Grand Hotel and cooled our heels for a couple of hours. I exchanged some texts with Mara and she didn't mention anything about a proposal, so I began wondering if Eric had lost his nerve or if he still had something up his sleeve. Soon it was time to get back in the limos for the actual Nobel Ceremony. Our motorcade drove the same one-mile distance to the Stockholm Concert Hall as we did earlier, but this time we drove much more slowly because there were massive crowds lining the sidewalk and cheering us on. Despite the bone-chilling temperatures, the crowd was at least five people deep the entire way, and the energy was unbelievable. Halfway there, my seat suddenly started vibrating. I asked our driver if he had turned on a massager, but he said he had not. I wondered if maybe I was hallucinating because I was so pumped with adrenaline from the roaring crowd. Ultimately, I discovered a toggle switch on the car door, which I must have accidently hit, so I was able to stop the vibrations.

There is nothing in the United States that compares to the Nobel Day events in Sweden. The best analogy would probably be Super Bowl weekend meets Oscar Night. December 10 is a national holiday in Sweden and TV coverage of the Nobel festivities is nonstop all day. Moreover, many Swedish citizens hold their own banquets in their houses and invite friends and relatives to dine and watch the Nobel Ceremony and Banquet together, sometimes in formal attire. Thus, many people from the huge crowd that was cheering us on would be heading to their Nobel dinner parties as soon as the motorcade passed.

When we arrived at the Concert Hall, I was ushered to the stage. In addition to the current class of Laureates, any Nobel Laureate who happens to be in town during the ceremony is invited to sit onstage. As it turned out, my close friends and fellow Yellow Berets Joe Goldstein and Mike Brown had spoken at the previous day's Nobel Symposium and stayed for the Nobel Ceremony. They were sitting right behind me, and it was amazing to share the experience with them. Forty years earlier, we had been hanging out in our tiny offices at the NIH, and now here we were dressed in white-tie tuxedos and sitting onstage together for the Nobel Ceremony. When my name was called, I strode across the stage to receive my medal from King Carl XVI Gustaf, feeling like I was walking on air.

Next up was the Nobel Banquet, held at the nearby Blue Hall in Stockholm City Hall. Everybody from the Nobel Ceremony had to be bused over to Blue Hall for the banquet. On the bus, I was approached by a Swedish journalist who was doing a television piece on what it takes to prepare for the Nobel Ceremony and Banquet.

"I want to interview you for this piece, Dr. Lefkowitz, because I've been asking around and everyone agrees that you're the happiest Laureate," she said.

Lynn cracked up when the journalist said this, and for the next several days teased me incessantly about my status as the "happiest Laureate." I had to admit, though, it was probably true. Brian was a natural introvert who was just trying to survive the onslaught of media attention; he couldn't wait to get out of the spotlight and back to his lab. Yamanaka was not a very happy Laureate either, as the ferocity of the Japanese paparazzi was making his life miserable. In contrast, I was having a ball.

I gave the reporter her interview and we headed inside Blue Hall for the Nobel Banquet. This banquet included more than 1,200 guests, all seated at tables around a central Table of Honor, which is where the Laureates sat along with their spouses, the royal family, and various government ministers. Everyone seated at the Table of Honor walked in last and had to descend down a long spiral staircase while the orchestra played. For this grand entrance, everyone at the Table of Honor was paired with another person of the opposite gender.

I was paired with Chika Yamanaka, the wife of Shinya Yamanaka. I found her to be a delightful woman—between our shared medical backgrounds (she is a dermatologist) and shared experiences of the past week, we had a lot to talk about. Chika had chosen to wear a kimono, the traditional dress of Japan, but her kimono had been pulled so tight by her assistant that she could barely move her legs. Moreover, there was a glaring discrepancy in our heights, so she needed to take several steps for every one of mine. At the top of the giant spiral staircase, we stopped to have a serious discussion about how exactly we were going to navigate the stairs together. I have to confess: I felt terrified that she was going to fall on the stairs, and perhaps take me down with her, so I resolved to do everything in my power to help avoid that scenario from happening. As the trumpets blared and we began our journey, I felt like a Sherpa helping a compromised mountain climber descend safely from a dangerous peak. When we reached the bottom, I exhaled deeply in relief at having avoided a potential disaster on the staircase.

The dinner service at the Nobel Banquet is unlike anything I have ever seen in my life. The menu and seating arrangements are published in advance, the entire event is televised, and the coverage is more intense than the coverage of the Oscars on American television. The Table of Honor consists of eighty people, who get served simultaneously by eighty different waiters. Hundreds of other waiters move in precision formation to serve the other tables, which seat more than 1,000 people. The food is amazing, and between courses there is entertainment, including musicians and acrobats. After dinner, there are brief speeches by the Laureates, with one Laureate from each category asked to say a few words. By tradition, the most senior Laureate in each category speaks, which worked out well in our case: I was more than happy to give the speech and Brian was thrilled *not* to give it.

When dinner was over and it was time for the speeches, a uniformed official led me from my seat up a set of stairs to a podium. I addressed my dinner companions with the following words:

"Your majesties, your royal highnesses, your excellences, ladies and gentleman,

To stand before this assembly as a Nobel Laureate, in the midst of these gala and festive surroundings, is simultaneously daunting, exhilarating, empowering, and most of all humbling. It is a remarkable moment, one to be savored. It is also a moment in which to feel a profound sense of gratitude. And on behalf of Brian Kobilka and myself, I would like to extend our heartfelt thanks to the Nobel Foundation for making all of this possible, and to the Royal Swedish Academy of Sciences for selecting us as the 2012 Nobel Laureates in Chemistry. Our gratitude extends as well to our collaborators and to the many dozens of students and fellows whose work in our laboratories is also honored by this award. We also thank our families, who are with us today, for their unflagging support of our often obsessive involvement with our work, especially our wives Tong Sung Kobilka and Lynn Lefkowitz. Tong Sung is not just Brian's wife, but she has also worked alongside him in the laboratory both as his technical assistant, dating back to his days in my laboratory more than twenty-five years ago, and for many years as his closest colleague and cheerleader, especially on his riskiest and most challenging projects.

No doubt, each Laureate's experience of receiving the Nobel Prize is unique. For me, one of the most poignant aspects relates to sharing this award with a former fellow of mine. I don't know how often a Nobel Prize is shared by a mentor and former trainee, but perusing the list of recent winners suggests that it is a reasonably common occurrence. This highlights an aspect of science that is very important to both Brian and me: the mentoring of young trainees. I have trained more than two hundred students and fellows in my lab over the past forty years, and a number of my and Brian's trainees have traveled to Stockholm to share this experience with us. They are in a very real sense a second family. Many of our trainees are major leaders in our field of science, a source of enormous pride for both of us.

But of course the annual award of the Nobel Prizes has significance that reaches far beyond the individual experiences of the Laureates. For those of us in the sciences, we watch with delight as every October the eyes of the entire world focus, if only transiently, on the power of discoveries in chemistry, physics, medicine, physiology, and economics to shape our lives. However, as an American scientist, and now Nobel Laureate, I have never been more aware or more appreciative of this effect of the prize announcements. We have just had a presidential election in the United States. One of the fault lines in the campaign was the role that science plays in shaping public policy decisions. A clear antiscience bias was apparent in many who sought the presidential nomination of one of our major political parties. This was manifest as a refusal to accept, for example, the theory of evolution, the existence of global warming, much less of the role of humans in this process, and the value of vaccines or of embryonic stem cell research. Each of us Laureates aspires in our own small way to do what we can to counter these pernicious antiscientific trends.

The work for which Brian and I are recognized today is the elucidation of the largest class of cellular receptors. These are the molecules on cells with which hormones, neurotransmitters, and other biologically active molecules interact, and they are the commonest target of therapeutic drugs such as opiates, beta blockers, and antihistamines, to mention just a few.

Our work lies at the ever-growing interface of chemistry and biology, a field generally referred to as biochemistry or biological chemistry, which is the chemistry of living things. In this context, it is of note that Brian and I both began our careers as physicians, and have ultimately traveled a long road to ever more fundamental research, one which has now led us to the Nobel Prize in Chemistry. To me it seems very much the fulfillment of an aspiration so beautifully expressed in a line from a poem entitled "Ithaca" by the Greek poet Constantine Cavafy, which has been taped above my desk for many, many years. It reads, *'When you set out on your journey to Ithaca, pray that the road is long, full of adventure, full of knowledge.'* I can tell you this . . . it certainly has been so far. Brian and I thank all of you for celebrating this journey with us."

The speech was well-received by the audience, and as I left the stage I could hear one of the television commentators providing commentary in an excited half-whisper: *"That was Dr. Robert Lefkowitz, Nobel Laureate in Chemistry, who really lit into the Republican Party in his home country . . ."* Of course, I had not said the word "Republican" in my remarks, and it was only one brief line in an eight-hundred-word speech, but nonetheless this comment ended up generating a fair amount of media attention.

When dinner was over, we moved next door to Golden Hall for cocktails and dancing. The king and queen were holding court in one corner of the room, and Lynn and I had a specific time slot for an audience with the royal family, from 11:30 to 11:40 P.M. We greatly enjoyed our brief chat with the king and queen and then sauntered back to our group, which included my kids along with other family members who had traveled to Stockholm for the occasion.

Suddenly, in an electric moment, Eric took Mara's hand and went down on one knee. Mara's reaction was priceless: she was literally slack-jawed, her mouth agape at Eric's gesture. My twelve-year-old grandson Jonah alertly whipped out his smartphone and began recording the proposal for the sake of posterity. Hundreds of people around us, who a moment earlier had been partying and carrying on their own conversations, went instantaneously silent and were riveted by the guy down on one knee offering a ring to my daughter. The king and queen were enthralled too, as Lynn and I had just left their company moments earlier. I saw the king craning his neck to get a better view of the commotion around us, and all of the other members of the royal family were also watching the proceedings with intense interest.

Mara tearfully accepted Eric's proposal. They embraced and kissed, which spurred the crowd around us to erupt into applause. One of the king's assistants hustled over and asked me for a clarification as to what had just happened; I told him that Eric had proposed marriage to my daughter Mara and she had accepted. The assistant ran back over to the king to relay the news, and the king's face lit up. He clasped his hands above his head and shook them back and forth in a triumphant gesture, which prompted the crowd to explode with applause a second time as they witnessed the king giving his blessing to Eric and Mara's union.

I couldn't stop smiling, first because I was so happy and second because of the irony of the situation. Two days earlier, Eric had vowed to propose to Mara in a low-key manner that would not attract attention. Somehow, he had ended up proposing to her right in front of the king and queen of Sweden, commanding their full attention with his dramatic gesture and creating a spectacle that was the talk of the Nobel Banquet. I was more than okay with his timing, though: the evening had already been special when I received my Nobel Medal, but now it was downright magical because I also had a new son-in-law who made my daughter so happy.

As the post-banquet reception slowed down, we headed out into the frigid night air to go to one of the after-parties organized by the students. Just like at the Oscars, there are numerous after-parties following the Nobel Banquet, and my entourage and I were not ready for the night to end. The after-party with the students was a blast, and then around 2:30 A.M. Lynn and I hopped back into our Nobel limo and headed back to the Grand Hotel. We got in a few hours of sleep but needed to be up at a respectable hour for an appointment at the Office of the Nobel Foundation to sign some documents and tend to certain administrative matters.[3]

When we woke up the next morning shortly after 8:00 A.M., we headed down to breakfast at the restaurant in the Grand Hotel. As we sat down at our table next to a large window, we saw two figures in disheveled tuxedos stumbling through the snow toward the Grand Hotel. I recognized them as Roger Sunahara and Yiorgo Skiniotis, two of Brian Kobilka's collaborators who had accompanied Brian to the Nobel festivities as his guests. They were just getting in at 8:30 A.M. after a long night of Nobel after-parties. I called them over to my table and asked for a full run-down on their nighttime exploits, then allowed them to head up to their rooms to crash on their beds. I envied their stamina but did not envy the rough shape they were in, as they looked like they were already paying the price for their marathon night of carousing and celebrating.

We were running on fumes ourselves, but the celebrations continued rolling full steam ahead. After our visit to the Office of the Nobel Foundation, I spent the afternoon at the Karolinska Institute for meetings with a few of the scientists there. Following that, it was time for another white-tie dinner: the Royal Banquet, hosted by the king and queen at the Royal Palace. This event was much smaller than the Nobel Banquet the previous evening, consisting of approximately 150 guests all seated at a single long table. Similar to the previous evening, dinner began with a procession in which everyone was paired off. This time, I was paired with Crown Princess Victoria, the heir to the Swedish throne. I strolled into the dining room with the princess on my arm and took my seat beside her.

Victoria was a most delightful dinner partner. I learned that she spoke four languages, had studied at both Uppsala University in Sweden and Yale University in the USA, and completed an internship in agriculture and forestry. She asked about my experience at the Nobel Banquet the previous night and I told her about Mara's surprise engagement, which caused the princess's eyes to well up with tears. She confessed to me that this story especially touched her due to the unusual circumstances of her own engagement: a few years earlier, she had fallen in love with her personal trainer, Daniel, who had then sought her father's blessing for marriage. However, the king did not give his blessing because Daniel was not of royal lineage. Victoria worked on her father over the course of many months and finally convinced him to give his blessing so that she could marry the man she loved. Given the difficult process of Victoria's own courtship and engagement, she was moved to hear how readily I had given my blessing and how excited I seemed to have Eric as part of my family.

After dinner, there was a champagne reception. I had the chance to schmooze with Prince Daniel, who I felt as though I already knew from chatting with his wife. Since Daniel had worked as a personal trainer, I talked with him about my own training regimen and he offered some helpful pointers. I also conversed with a number of other interesting people at the reception, but eventually began to flag from staying out so late the night before. I was told that it was against protocol to retire for the evening until the king retired, so I found a Swedish colleague of mine and made a covert inquiry.

"When will this thing finish?"

"Well," my Swedish friend replied. "Certainly not before the king finishes his cigar."

From that point forward, I watched the king's cigar intensely as he smoked it down. When he finally snuffed it out, I felt a sense of relief and downed my last gulp of champagne. I was just about to grab Lynn and tell her to get ready to go when suddenly the king grabbed another stogie out of an ornate humidor presented to him by an aide and lit it up. I sighed, grabbed another flute of champagne, and girded myself for another hour or two of partying.

The next day, I traveled to a high school on the outskirts of Stockholm. One of the most wonderful traditions of Nobel Week is that the Laureates get invited to many local schools and universities to interact with the students. It's impossible to accept all the invitations, of course, but it's fun to accept a few of them. At the high school, I gave a brief talk and then signed a few hundred autographs for the students, including one for a young lady who requested to have her forehead signed.

"When will you wash it off?" I asked.

"Not any time soon!" she answered enthusiastically.

The day after the high school visit, Lynn and I traveled to Uppsala University, the alma mater of Crown Princess Victoria. I gave a talk there, signed more autographs, and had lunch with some of the students. Memorably, the student who drove us on the one-hour ride from Stockholm to Uppsala told us that his parents were reindeer farmers. I asked him what it was like to grow up on a reindeer farm and he launched into a fascinatingly detailed description of the finer points of raising reindeer.

I had so much fun on these student visits that I could've stayed in Sweden for several more weeks. The whole trip had been like a fairy tale, and I didn't want to see it end. However, I had a flight to catch and a life back home to which I was eager to return. I was thinking that things would just return to normal after I got home. What I had not yet realized, though, was just how dramatically my life would be changed now that I had received the Nobel Prize.

TWENTY-THREE

The New Normal

After our plane touched down back in the United States, Lynn and I collected our bags and exited the airport to find a ride home.

"Hey, where's our limo?" I asked in mock confusion. It's amazing how rapidly a personal car and chauffeur can start to feel like a birthright. The fairy tale in Sweden was over, though, so I had to hail a cab like normal.

Indeed, some things in my life remained completely normal after winning the Nobel Prize. My relationships with Lynn and my kids were unchanged. My interactions with the trainees in my lab were exactly the same, and overall my day-to-day schedule was not much different. However, other things in my life were *very* different, and rapidly I realized that I would need to get adjusted to a new post-Nobel definition of "normal."

For starters, my email inbox was flooded with messages, many of the bizarre variety. In my pre-Nobel life, I had been invited to many conferences, but usually to meetings in my areas of expertise, such as receptors or cardiology. As a Nobel Laureate, though, I was now receiving scores of invitations to speak on topics I knew nothing about, including nano-technology, gynecology, world peace, and the nature of consciousness. It is true that many Nobel Laureates *do* begin broadcasting their opinions on every topic under the sun, as if winning a Nobel Prize somehow confers boundless knowledge in all fields, but in my case I did not sense I had experienced any sudden surge in wisdom. Thus, the invitations I received to conferences about extraterrestrial intelligence and other topics in which I was not well-versed went straight into the trash.

Certain requests did attract my attention. In particular, I reveled in the many invitations I received to speak at local schools. I love speaking to young people to convey my passion for research and learning, so I accepted as many such invitations as I possibly could. When I was a youngster, I would've been thrilled to meet a Nobel Laureate at school, especially a Nobel Laureate who was a physician, but I never had the opportunity. Thus, in the first few years after I won the Nobel, I gave numerous talks at grade schools, middle schools, and high schools, enjoying every single one of these events. Along the same lines, I also accepted an invitation from an organization called the American Academy of Achievement.

This organization was founded in 1961 by Brian Blaine Reynolds, a photographer for *Life* magazine who wanted to help young people meet high achievers to hear their inspiring stories. The goal of these meetings is to help transfer knowledge from one generation to the next and promote the development of the next wave of thought leaders. I attended the 2014 meeting in San Francisco, where I received my Golden Plate (the symbol of induction into the Academy) from Francis Collins, the director of the National Institutes of Health and former leader of the Human Genome Project. Other honorees being inducted that year included Diana Ross, Carol Burnett, Sydney Poitier, Chef Thomas Keller, Admiral William McRaven (of Navy SEAL fame), and my fellow Nobelists Louis Ignarro and Frances Arnold. It was fun to rub shoulders with these giants and even more fun to interact with all the enthusiastic students at this event.

I also attended the next Academy of Achievement Summit in 2017 in London and had another great time. Now that I was a member, I had the honor of giving out a Golden Plate to Brian Kobilka as he joined the academy. At the reception after the induction ceremony, I was approached by Peter Gabriel and Sting, who were being inducted for their songwriting genius and humanitarian efforts. Peter had a medical question, which I quickly answered, and then we continued chatting for a while. I mentioned that my son David worked in the music industry as a manager, and Lynn suggested that we should take a photo and text it to David. As Lynn got the camera ready, Peter said to Sting, *"We should kneel down to show his son how much we worship him."* Before I knew it, both Peter and Sting were kneeling before me as Lynn snapped a photo. This moment was a clear example of how winning a Nobel Prize changed my life: pre-Nobel, I had received a modicum of recognition within the scientific community, but post-Nobel I underwent a quantum leap in celebrity status, leading to outlandish situations such as having two of the greatest songwriters of all time kneeling before me in a show of faux adulation.

In addition to invitations to conferences,[1] I also received a number of offers for honorary degrees. The honorary degree that generated by far the most media attention was the one I received from the Baylor College of Medicine. I began tracking my mentions in the media using Google Alerts because of previous issues I'd had with being misquoted or cited incorrectly, as described in earlier chapters; I learned the hard way that if I am misquoted somewhere, it's best to address the problem right away rather than waiting. In any case, after I accepted the invitation to receive an honorary degree at Baylor, my Google Alerts began blowing up with numerous mentions of my name in the popular media. Naturally, this made me curious as to why my honorary degree from Baylor was attracting such attention.

It turned out that the football player J. J. Watt was to blame. The star defensive end for the Houston Texans was also receiving an honorary degree from Baylor and generating an enormous amount of media buzz for philanthropic work he was doing to help flood victims in Houston. Every article published about J. J. noted that he was set to receive an honorary degree from Baylor, with the next line in the article saying something like, "Also receiving an honorary degree is Robert Lefkowitz, Nobel Laureate from Duke." Thus, all the popular articles featuring my name weren't really about me, but rather were about J. J. and his efforts to help flood victims.

I told this story to J. J. while we were having dinner together after the Baylor graduation ceremony and we shared a laugh about it. J. J. is possibly the largest human I've ever met, a true modern-day Paul Bunyan: 6' 5" and 300 pounds of pure muscle. He had to leave dinner immediately after polishing off his entree because he was getting up at an insanely early hour the next day to start his summer football practices with the Texans. I felt happy to share the Baylor graduation honor with J. J., as I saw in him a man completely dedicated to his craft as well as a philanthropist who gave an enormous amount of his time to those in need.

Another sports icon who I had the good fortune to spend time with during this period was Mike Krzyzewski, the head coach of the Duke basketball team. As mentioned in an earlier chapter, I first met Coach K after the Nobel Prize announcement when he called me with congratulations and arranged for me to be honored at Cameron Indoor Stadium. Subsequently, we ended up spending time together at a number of Duke events, including leadership seminars that the coach runs and various celebrations on the Duke campus, such as when my colleague Paul Modrich became the second Nobel Laureate from Duke in late 2015.

Earlier that year, Coach K had led Duke to the school's fifth national championship in men's basketball. The team was invited by President

Obama to visit the White House, where they presented Obama with a Duke #1 jersey. When I saw this event on the news, I immediately took a photo of *my* Duke #1 jersey, which was hanging in my office, and emailed it to Coach K along with a note that read:

"Dear Mike, I was excited that the team won the national title again and pleased that President Obama invited you to the White House. However, couldn't you have given Obama a different jersey number? As you can see in the attached photo, the Duke #1 jersey was raised to the rafters after you gave it to me, so the number is retired!"

Within the hour, Coach K replied back to me with his usual humor and tact.

"Bob, you are right! We should have gotten your permission before we gave it to him! You are the real #1 and always will be."

In addition to having my Duke jersey number given away to Obama, I also suffered a number of other indignities as a result of my newfound celebrity status. Notably, I was portrayed as a drug- and sex-crazed jerk on *The Late Show with David Letterman.*

"In our audience tonight, we have one of the winners of the 2012 Nobel Prize in Chemistry," Letterman said after his monologue one evening. "Do me a favor, please welcome Robert J. Lefkowitz!"

The audience cheered, and a guy who looked nothing like me stood up in the fourth row and waved. He was wearing a gold medal around his neck.

"Sir, it's good to have you here," Dave solemnly intoned. "Thank you on behalf of the nation and the world. What are your plans now that you've won the Nobel Prize?"

"Well," the guy said. "After the show, I'm gonna go back to the hotel and get me a cheeseburger and some weed."

The camera returned to Dave, who had a bemused look on this face. He then asked a question of the audience.

"How many of you are gonna do that tonight?"

The audience erupted with wild applause. The members of the band all raised their hands as well, prompting Dave to shout, *"You guys aren't even staying at a hotel!"*

Several minutes later, Dave interrupted his next bit to make an announcement.

"I'm being told that the 2012 Nobel Laureate in Chemistry, Dr. Robert Lefkowitz, has something else to say. Yes, doctor?"

The guy stood up again.

"Dave, I forgot to mention: after the cheeseburger and the weed, I'm gonna get laid. Who's with me?" Naturally, the audience went crazy again.

"I don't think that's really the Nobel Prize winner," Dave said when the camera returned to him. Finally, a few minutes later, "Dr. Lefkowitz" raised his hand one last time. He stood up, revealing the gold medal was no longer around his neck.

"Yes doctor, what is it now?" asked Dave.

"The Nobel Committee found out about the weed, and they took my prize away. Thanks a lot, asshole!"

Shortly after this episode aired, I was speaking on the phone with Brian Kobilka and he mentioned he saw it. He thought the bit was very disrespectful, and expected I would feel the same. I told Brian that in truth I found the bit hilarious. My only regret was that Letterman didn't fly me in to play myself, as I was convinced I could've delivered the lines better than the actor playing me.

❖

Beyond invitations to conferences and offers of honorary degrees, my post-Nobel life also featured other sorts of opportunities that had not been afforded to me prior to winning the Nobel Prize. For example, in 2013, shortly after I won the prize, I was invited to throw out ceremonial first pitches at two different baseball games: a Durham Bulls game in Durham, North Carolina, and a New York Yankees game in New York City. The Yankees game was especially meaningful, as I had grown up as a Yankees fan and attended many games at the old Yankee Stadium during my childhood.

I hadn't thrown a baseball in years, so I decided I needed to practice before tossing these pitches in front of thousands of fans. A month before the Yankees game, I went out into the backyard with Lynn and measured out 60 feet, 6 inches, the distance of a major league mound from home plate.

"Holy cow," I said to Lynn, who was holding the tape measure at the starting point to assist with the measurement. I shaded my eyes against the slant of the afternoon sun. Lynn was so faraway that it looked like I was viewing her through the wrong end of a telescope. "This looks a little farther than I thought."

I proceeded to toss a few dozen pitches, with Lynn serving as my catcher. My first few throws were embarrassingly short. I ramped up the power to gain more distance, but this caused me to become wild, forcing Lynn to run all over the yard retrieving my errant heaves. I realized that I was going to need more practice to avoid looking bad while throwing out these ceremonial pitches.

The students and postdocs in my lab were highly amused by my anxiety over these first pitch invitations and spent the next few weeks trying to psych me out. Every day, I would arrive at my office, open my email, and find yet another video compilation of the "Top 10 Worst Ceremonial First Pitches of All Time." I have to admit, these videos spooked me. Perhaps the worst was when I encountered Harrison Ford in my inbox. There stood Indiana Jones, a guy who seemed like a pretty good athlete, but even he threw from the mound with an awkward motion, bouncing the ball far in front of home plate. There was another video of a guy falling off the mound and tumbling head over heels while winding up for a first pitch, and yet another clip of a guy who was so wild that he somehow threw the ball 20 feet to the left of home plate and hit one of the umpires in the head.

After viewing these videos, I decided that I needed to get some serious coaching. During a business trip to San Francisco, I added an extra day to my itinerary in order to consult with my granddaughter Maya, a star pitcher on her high school softball team. When I showed her my pitching motion, she shook her head in dismay and told me that I lacked power because I was throwing sidearm. She then patiently reconfigured my delivery so that I was throwing overhand, resulting in a massive gain in my throwing power. A few weeks later, during a family beach vacation attended by most of my kids and grandchildren, I spent many hours playing catch with Maya and receiving additional instruction.

Back at Duke, I began having daily throwing sessions with the trainees from my lab. At lunchtime, we would bring our baseball gloves down to a courtyard adjacent to our building and play catch for twenty minutes. Unexpectedly, these sessions began attracting large numbers of spectators, with scientists from nearby labs gathering to watch the Nobel Laureate toss the ol' baseball around with the members of his lab. People would just sit at nearby picnic tables, eat their sandwiches, and watch us throw. They probably thought we were doing it as some kind of team-building exercise, but in fact I was focused on building up my arm strength. I have to admit, though, these sessions did create a sense of lab bonding, with everyone in the lab coming together to help the boss get ready to take the mound. Perhaps they didn't want me to embarrass them, either!

As the date for the Yankees game approached, I received some bad news: I was getting bumped from throwing out the first pitch. The game for which I had been tentatively scheduled was the first visit to New York by the Boston Red Sox after the Boston Marathon bombing incident, so the Yankees were planning a pregame ceremony to honor the victims of this terrorist event. As part of the ceremony, they wanted someone connected to fighting terrorism to throw out the first pitch, which led them to invite former New York City Mayor Rudy Giuliani in place of me. I understood the rationale, but nonetheless was disappointed to miss the opportunity, especially since there was no follow-up by the Yankees to reschedule my first pitch for a later game.

Even though the Yankees game went by the boards, I was still looking forward to throwing out the first pitch at the Durham Bulls game. The week before the game, I decided that the final step in my preparation needed to be throwing off an actual pitching mound. I explained the situation to the pitching coach of the Duke baseball team, Andrew See, and he invited me to throw some pitches off the mound at Duke's baseball stadium one afternoon. I was accompanied by my postdoc Jeff Kovacs, who served as my catcher, and several members of the Duke baseball coaching staff, who gave me helpful pointers to avoid falling off the mound or plunking umpires in the head. After all of this coaching and preparation, I felt like I was ready to go.

The pregame festivities at the Durham Bulls ballpark were quite a scene. The mayor of Durham, Bill Bell, read a proclamation declaring it "Robert Lefkowitz Week," and Victor Dzau, the president and chief executive officer of the Duke University Health System, said a few brief words about my research. Then it was time for me to take the mound.[2] I strode out to the pitching rubber, went into a big windup featuring a full leg kick, and then fired a perfect strike to home plate. The crowd, which included all the members of my laboratory, went bananas. The catcher trotted out to hand the ball back to me, patting me on the back as he spoke.

"Doc, that was one helluva throw!"

As fun as it was to be honored at baseball games and other events, I still found my greatest joy during this period in the more normal parts of my schedule: spending time in the lab talking about data and traveling to give seminars about my lab's latest studies, which were increasingly becoming focused on applying the biophysical approaches that Brian and his collaborators had developed to address questions about how receptors interact with beta-arrestins.[3] After winning the Nobel Prize, I got invited to speak everywhere and could only accept a small fraction of the invitations, but I never turned down requests from former trainees. Whenever an alum from my lab wanted me to come speak, I always found a way to make it happen. With each passing year, I felt prouder and prouder of my scientific family tree, and spent more and more time reflecting on what it means to be a mentor.

TWENTY-FOUR

The Art of Mentoring

The most meaningful part of my professional career has come from mentoring young scientists and watching them develop. I have mentored more than two hundred trainees, with a large percentage of them going on to enjoy highly successful careers in academia or industry. Many have won major research awards, and one has even received the Nobel Prize. Due to this track record, I have often been asked: How do you do it? What is your secret formula for producing generation after generation of standout scientists?

For many years, I was flummoxed by such questions. I had no secret formula for mentoring. In fact, in my first two decades running my own lab, I hardly thought about mentoring at all. Yogi Berra, the legendary Yankees catcher, was once asked what he thought about while batting, and his response was, *"How ya gonna think and hit at the same time?"* That was exactly how I felt about mentoring. I wasn't thinking about it,

I was just doing research and trying to exhort the students in my lab to come along on the journey with me.

Over the years, though, I have become more mindful about my mentoring approach. I have learned a lot from my mentoring successes, as well as my mentoring failures, and accumulated a lifetime's worth of wisdom in this area. I am not so presumptuous as to believe that I have discovered the One True Way of Mentoring, but I know what works for me. After a half century spent mentoring hundreds of trainees, here are my ten golden rules for being a good mentor:

1. *Tailor mentoring to each individual's needs.* Every trainee is different. Some need a daily pat on the shoulder, some need a kick in the pants. For this reason, I have always customized my mentoring style to each individual who joins my group. Sometimes this means shifting my approach around for a while until I find what works for each person. Obviously, such custom-tailoring of mentoring style requires getting to know the members of my lab very well, which is why I view daily chitchat as not simply an exchange of pleasantries, but instead as a crucial opportunity to get to know my junior colleagues' personal stories and understand what motivates and excites them.

Every individual has strengths and weaknesses. My goal as a mentor is to emphasize the strengths while mitigating the weaknesses. If I am working with a young scientist who is very creative but doesn't pay much attention to detail, it's probably not going to help if I constantly badger them about becoming more detail oriented. That's just going to make us both miserable. In my experience, it is more productive with such a trainee to emphasize their strength, by praising and encouraging their creativity, while at the same time trying to mitigate their weakness, perhaps by pairing them with a collaborator who by nature is more detail-conscious but perhaps lacks that creative spark. I am not above the occasional gentle prompt in an area that needs work, but it's important to realize you are not going to change someone's fundamental nature.

Mentoring should be tailored not just to each individual mentee but also to the personality of the mentor. The specific strategies that work for me as a mentor might not work for someone else. For example, I am a very social and gregarious person. I love face-to-face meetings and crave constant contact with the members of my group. However, I know some scientists who are much more reserved, but nonetheless are still great mentors. They might prefer regular communication with their trainees via e-mail or other written forms of communication, as opposed to having a large number of face-to-face meetings. Every mentor has to find the specific approaches that work for them, which is why I have crafted the remaining nine precepts below as general guidelines rather than detailed rules.

2. *Encourage focus.* Whenever any new trainee joins my group, I meet with them on their first day and give them two pieces of advice. The first piece of advice is: *"Your success in my laboratory will be determined by four factors: the first is focus, the second is focus, the third is focus, and the fourth is . . . focus."* In research, as in any creative endeavor, there are countless directions in which an ambitious young person might proceed. I view my primary job as helping my trainees focus on productive and interesting directions. Everything else is secondary to focus.

When I was a medical student, I had an old microscope that I'd purchased for a pittance from an older student who no longer needed it. I used this microscope in my classes and also in my dorm room to study for exams. This ancient microscope was so beat up that the stage was always slipping, which would cause the scope to drift out of focus every few seconds. Over time, I became skilled at holding the microscope in focus by keeping my fingers on the fine-tuning knob and exerting just the right amount of pressure. Many years later, I realized that my most crucial job as a mentor is to manage my trainees in the same way I managed my old medical school microscope: by constantly exerting just the right amount of pressure to keep things in focus.

Whenever I travel for a week, I find upon my return that certain projects in the lab have drifted out of focus. Perhaps there was a surprising finding that led a trainee down a side road, resulting in a series of unplanned experiments. Sometimes side roads can lead to new discoveries, but more commonly they just lead to dead ends. When I return from travel and talk with a student who is spinning their wheels in a dead end, I'll say, *"Let's remember the big-picture goal of this project. How is what you're doing right now helping to reach that goal?"* Through discussion along these lines, the student will usually realize they've lost focus and gotten distracted by insignificant details. My aim in such conversations is to gently exert the right amount of pressure on the fine-tuning knob to keep the student in focus, just like I used to do with my old microscope.

3. *Fan the flames of enthusiasm.* The second piece of advice that I give to new members of my lab on their first day is, *"You can work on any project you want, as long as two conditions are met: the first is that you should be very excited about your project, and the second is that I should be very excited about your project."* Those two conditions are not sufficient for a given project to succeed, but they are necessary. Research is 90 percent failure, so it's easy for students to get down when their project isn't going well. A critical role for mentors is to keep trainees pumped up so they can make it through the hard times and maintain their focus.

Many years after my postdoc Rick Cerione headed off to Cornell University to direct his own research group, he confided to me that during his time in my lab he felt like he was working on the most important project in the lab. However, when he talked to other folks in the lab at that time, he realized that each of them also believed that *they* were working on the most important project in the lab. In Rick's telling, I was somehow able to convince every single person in my group that they were working on the most important project in the history of science. In truth, when I was talking with each of those folks about their experiments in the early days of my lab, I probably did believe in the moment that each project was the most important one. I wasn't faking it—I was authentically psyched up and conveyed this passion to my students in a way that fanned the flames of their enthusiasm. Such shared delusions of grandeur between mentor and trainee can be very powerful motivators for young scientists and may lead to achievements beyond what they believed possible.

Enthusiasm is a critical trait shared by all great mentors, but it's important to point out that there *is* such a thing as too much enthusiasm. In my early days as a faculty member, I heard stories about a well-known scientist at the University of California San Francisco (UCSF). He was famous for roaming through his lab and getting excited about everything. Even if a student were just performing a mundane task, like adjusting the pH of a buffer, this scientist would exclaim, *"Wow! Look at that! You got the pH to exactly 7.0! Fantastic job!!!"* In my view, constant praise of this sort is counterproductive. It cheapens the value of the mentor's enthusiasm, which should be reserved for truly worthy efforts. Trainees can sense when their mentor is manufacturing enthusiasm versus feeling authentically excited, and they only respond to the latter.

Enthusiasm needs to be balanced with rigor. My first two mentors, Jesse Roth and Ira Pastan, represented the personification of these two ideals. As described in an earlier chapter, Jesse was Mr. Enthusiasm. He didn't necessarily get excited about adjusting the pH of buffers like the scientist at UCSF, but he would ooh and aah over just about any piece of data I showed him. In contrast, Ira almost never got excited. When I showed him data, he would just grill me over whether I had included the appropriate controls. Off the top of his head, Ira could name ten different reasons why any given result might be a complete artifact. Years later, when I became a mentor myself, I did my best to combine Jesse's enthusiasm with Ira's rigor. Trainees need both of those ingredients to thrive.

4. *Teach trainees to build their careers around problems, not techniques.* Sometimes trainees learn a new technique and then spend the next few months or years, or in some cases their entire careers, looking for other problems to which they can apply their newly learned technique over and over again. This is exactly the wrong approach for developing a career in science, or indeed in any creative field. Techniques are always changing as new technologies evolve. Thus, mentors should advise their trainees to ask big-picture questions about important problems, and then try to answer those questions using whatever techniques are necessary.

Joe Goldstein, my friend and fellow Yellow Beret, wrote an outstanding essay on this topic many years ago.[1] Joe coined the term PAIDS, which stands for "Paralyzed Academic Investigator's Disease Syndrome." This condition occurs when a scientist learns a narrow set of techniques and then becomes limited to only asking questions that can be addressed with those techniques. Joe also coined another term I love, "technical courage," which is the fearlessness exhibited by scientists who choose to work on an important problem and commit themselves to learning whatever techniques are necessary to address that problem. One of the most crucial things mentors can do is to model technical courage and push their trainees to be bold in learning new techniques and adopting new technologies.

Brian Kobilka has exemplified technical courage throughout his career. When Brian first joined my lab, he was a cardiology fellow who knew very few research techniques. However, he sensed that the identification of the genes encoding the beta-adrenergic receptors (and other receptors) was the next important step to be taken in the field, so he dedicated himself to learning the new molecular biology techniques that were emerging at that time. Years later, when Brian was directing his own lab at Stanford, he sensed that the next big problem was to elucidate the three-dimensional structure of the receptors, so he spent a decade learning the art of X-ray crystallography and encouraging his students to be similarly fearless in mastering the emerging techniques of the structural biology field. Brian is an exceptional mentor to his students because he doesn't just preach technical courage, he models it every single day.

5. *Promote risk-taking.* When students take laboratory classes in school, they usually perform cookbook experiments with known outcomes. In such prefabricated experiments, you are supposed to get a certain result, and if you get a different result then it means you screwed up. However, true scientific research is the opposite: if you get a result you didn't expect, it's often a sign that you're onto an interesting story. Pursuing ideas that cut against existing paradigms seems risky to many trainees, though, which is why mentors must encourage boldness when projects start moving into uncharted waters. I teach all my trainees the Yiddish term "chutzpah," which loosely means "brazen audacity." Every great researcher needs to possess some degree of chutzpah.

Researchers who are afraid to take risks will never reach their full potential. I had dinner once with a researcher in the visual signaling field who said he had made a significant discovery about the visual receptor rhodopsin some years earlier. The finding was so unexpected that he had doubts about it and was afraid to publish it because others would doubt it as well. He dawdled and pursued various tangential studies, feeling uncertain how to proceed. Eventually, two other labs published his novel finding before he did, so he got scooped and received no credit for his big discovery. This was a classic case of a scientist who would have benefited from a mentor who encouraged more chutzpah.

Promoting risk-taking does not mean that mentors should encourage their trainees to go on wild-goose chases. Mentors should encourage their young charges to maintain a balanced portfolio of related projects, with some directions being straightforward and other directions being riskier but with potentially bigger payoffs. Each year around the holidays, I perform an annual review of every research direction in my lab, and when I'm done I compare my notes to those from previous years. One year, a colleague walked into my office while I was performing this end-of-year analysis. When I explained what I was doing, he began to enthuse about the great year his lab had just completed.

"Yeah, I'd say about 90 percent of my lab's projects this year worked out," he said with a satisfied smile. "How about you?"

"Well, according to my analysis, about 20 percent of my lab's research directions this year yielded fruit," I replied. "The other 80 percent have thus far flamed out."

My colleague's jaw dropped.

"I'm actually thrilled with that number," I continued. "If the percentage of successful projects in my lab gets too close to 50 percent, then it means we're not taking enough risks."

6. *Model dogged persistence.* Success in any competitive field requires hard work. As mentioned above, success rates for cutting-edge research experiments are quite low. Thus, the best way to achieve success is to do a *lot* of experiments. Eventually, something will work and lead to exciting new directions. However, it's insufficient to tell trainees they need to work hard to succeed. Actions speak louder than words, so it's crucial for mentors to serve as role models of dogged persistence.

I became a Howard Hughes investigator in 1976. Every five years after that, as described in an earlier chapter, I had to renew my appointment via a rigorous process that involved writing about the work my lab had done and then giving a talk in front of a Howard Hughes panel. I always began preparing for these presentations months in advance. I would ask various trainees in my group to help prepare slides, and then work through multiple drafts of each slide until they were just right. When the slides were ready, I would give a series of practice talks, sometimes by myself and sometimes in front of small groups of trainees from my lab. The hard work on the slides and practice talks prepared me well for my renewal presentations. However, these efforts also served another purpose: they showed my trainees how hard I was working to make my presentations shine. The unspoken message was that I also expected my trainees to work hard on *their* presentations, whether they were preparing for a lab meeting, job talk, or platform presentation at a national conference.

There are many ways to model a strong work ethic. Whenever one of my trainees sends me a rough draft of a manuscript to be submitted for publication, I make every effort to send the edited manuscript back to them with the fastest turnaround time possible. If one of my trainees needs a letter of recommendation, then *boom*, I get it done as fast as I possibly can. Fast turnaround times show my trainees that I give them high priority, and also send the message that I expect equally fast turnaround times on their end. I have heard stories about mentors who try to push their trainees by keeping track of the number of hours people are working or other such nonsense. To me, such approaches are ineffective and will only lead to trainees feeling stressed out. The best way for mentors to encourage persistence and hard work is simply to model such behavior themselves.

7. *Empower trainees.* People achieve their maximum level of motivation when they feel ownership over their work. For this reason, I want every person in my lab to feel like they are pursuing their own ideas, as opposed to working on a project cooked up by me or someone else. When I have weekly meetings with my trainees, I never say to them, *"Well, based on these data, you should next do this and then do that."* Instead, I ask what new directions *they* would find interesting to pursue. When I hear a direction that excites me, I say something like, *"Wow, yes, that would be*

interesting to explore, wouldn't it?" In this way, my trainees are driving their own projects, and my role is simply to serve as guide and cheerleader.

I know some scientific mentors who create daily to-do lists for the members of their labs. I'll admit to being impressed with anyone who has the brainpower to write out detailed schedules for a lab full of scientists every day, but to me this is still an example of ineffective mentoring. When trainees are micromanaged in this manner, they lack a sense of ownership over their projects, decreasing their motivation and also stunting their growth as independent thinkers. Inevitably, mentors who micromanage produce few if any trainees who later achieve success as principal investigators, as those trainees were never allowed to spread their intellectual wings during their training period and thus didn't learn how to develop projects. Moreover, even when such micromanaged trainees make good progress under their mentor's close guidance, they never develop the confidence that comes from knowing that they were truly the ones responsible for their own success.

8. *Emphasize storytelling.* I received an early lesson in the importance of storytelling from one of my clinical mentors, Mortimer Bader. As described in an earlier chapter, Bader was an attending physician at Mount Sinai Hospital who was legendary for challenging medical students to come up with different narratives that would fit the facts of a given clinical case.

"Many people think data tell a story, but nothing could be further from the truth," Bader would say. "Data are just data. A *story* is something you impose on the data."

Bader's insight was crucial to my development as a clinician and even more critical to my eventual evolution as a scientist. When I have meetings with my trainees, I don't just want them to show me their data: I also want to hear a story that explains the data. Ideally, I want my students to present *multiple* stories that might explain the data, and then propose future studies that will help to discern which narrative is closer to the truth.

In addition to its importance in making sense of experiments on a day-to-day basis, storytelling is also important to a mentor over years and decades. I want my trainees to feel like they are key players in an ongoing story, which began long ago and has continued for many years with numerous twists and turns. The feeling that you are part of something larger than yourself is one of the most powerful human emotions, especially when you feel like you are contributing to a narrative arc that stretches far back in time. For this reason, I love telling my trainees stories about earlier generations in my lab and how certain studies performed back in the day connect with experiments that are currently ongoing. This feeling of a cohesive narrative through the years is very motivating for trainees, who feel excited to understand how their current experiments fit into the grand scheme of research in the field.

9. *Laugh and have fun.* Humor is a great prod to creativity. In my experience, the more people are laughing, the more creative they become. This may be due to the fact that humor requires seeing unusual connections between things. "Getting" a joke is like making a little discovery: you have a flash of insight and suddenly see a funny connection that you didn't previously see. The creativity required for humor can prime the mind for other sorts of creativity. For this reason, I am constantly joking around in meetings with my trainees, with the humorous tone hopefully setting the stage for inspiration.

A few years ago, I had a conference call with a pharmaceutical company about a potential collaboration. I was on the call with four young postdoctoral fellows from my lab at Duke, and we were talking with four or five scientists from the company. The leader of the company's scientific team started off the call.

"Okay Professor Lefkowitz, let me introduce my team. We have here Carlos, who is our director of Chemistry, and Nina, who's our director of Molecular Screening . . ."

When I heard these introductions, I decided on the spot that I was not going to be outdone. The four young postdocs from my lab didn't have any titles—they were just postdocs. However, the pharmaceutical company folks on the other end of the call didn't know that. When it was my turn to speak, I ad-libbed a series of introductions.

"Great, thank you, now I'll introduce my team. I've got here Erin, who is our director of protein purification, and Scott, our director of mass spectrometry . . ."

As I was making the introductions, my trainees began cracking up as I gave them fancy-sounding titles. Fortunately, it was a regular phone call, not a video conference, so the people on the other end of the call couldn't see all my postdocs trying to stifle their laughter. It was a funny moment, and it led to a productive conference call with lots of creative ideas being tossed around by the members of my group.

Humor is also important because it creates an enjoyable work environment. If your job feels like nonstop drudgery, it's difficult to work long hours. It's much easier to put in those hours if your work feels like play. I have always tried to maintain a playful attitude in my lab, including placing bets with trainees about how experiments will come out and offering fun prizes when certain milestones are accomplished. For example, when my lab succeeded in completing the sequencing of the beta-2 adrenergic receptor gene, I offered my team a limo ride to lunch at the restaurant of their choice. The team included Brian and Tong Sun Kobilka, Tom Frielle, Henrik Dohlman, and a few others. On the way back from lunch, they stopped at McDonald's just for the sheer comic value of taking a limo to the drive-through window to order a round of milkshakes. It was a great moment of lab bonding that also helped to maintain a playful attitude at a time when many members of the lab were putting in long hours.

10. *Respect your own mentors.* Everyone needs mentoring, even seasoned mentors. For this reason, it's important to maintain strong relationships

with past mentors, such that they can serve as sounding boards for any mentoring problems or career issues that might arise. Over the years, I have sought out my mentor Jesse Roth at national meetings, or sometimes just called him out of the blue, to discuss various issues and listen to his perspectives. In turn, many of my alumni who are now established mentors in their own right call me regularly to talk through various issues relating to their research groups. In my view, mentoring is not something you do just for a couple of years while someone is working with you; the position of mentor is a lifetime appointment, much like being a parent. I am always delighted to catch up with my past trainees and provide whatever insights I can to help them at different stages of their careers.

I am old enough now to have hundreds of scientific children (i.e., former trainees from my lab) and probably thousands of scientific grandchildren and great-grandchildren (i.e., the trainees of my trainees). When I attend meetings these days, I love schmoozing with members of my scientific family. I derive a great deal of pleasure from seeing all the exciting work my trainees are pursuing and the ways in which they are passing on the torch to the next generation of scientists. Many scientific meetings in my field feel like family reunions of former trainees, which reminds me of the joy I derive from spending time with my actual family, especially at large gatherings such as our annual yearly reunion at the beach. I have always been a family man, and several recent events have led me to an even deeper connection to my family's legacy than I could have previously imagined.

TWENTY-FIVE

Roots

I was hiking deep in the woods near Czestochowa, Poland, and beginning to worry that our guide had gotten us lost. I was accompanied by Lynn, my cousins Ellen and Judy, and Judy's husband, Ivan. Supposedly, we were looking for my family's roots, but I doubted we were going to find them this far out in this forest.

I had taken this trip to Poland with Lynn and my cousins in 2017 because I had been invited to speak at the Polish Academy of Sciences. It was my first trip ever to Poland, so I decided to add a few extra days to the trip to spend more time learning about my family's ancestral home. My paternal grandparents emigrated from Poland to the USA in 1904. They were fleeing the pogroms (organized massacres of Jewish people) that were happening in Eastern Europe at that time. My father was born in New York City in 1905, which means he might have been in utero with my grandmother when she was on the run.

The suffering of the European Jews of this era has always been personal to me. During my trip to Poland with Lynn and my cousins, we toured various sites related to the Holocaust. This included the infamous concentration camps at Auschwitz and Birkenau. The horrors that went on there are frankly beyond imagining, and the tour was emotionally draining. We also toured Oskar Schindler's factory, which is now a museum. In this factory, Schindler saved 1,200 Polish Jews from the Holocaust by employing them and bribing Nazi officials to look the other way; this story is the basis for the movie *Schindler's List*. The Schindler museum in Krakow has a wall listing all the people who Schindler protected, and eight or nine of these names are the Polish spelling of "Lefkowitz." There's a good chance that some of these people were my relatives. Similarly, at the Holocaust Museum in Washington, D.C., there are many thick volumes listing alphabetically all the lives lost in the Holocaust, and numerous pages in these books are dedicated to the various spellings of the name "Lefkowitz." There seems little doubt that some of those folks were my kin.

In advance of the Poland trip, we hired a team of local document detectives to hunt down information relating to my family. They uncovered a trove of birth certificates, marriage certificates, and other documents from my family's past, and also were able to locate my grandparents' old house in Czestochowa, a small town about 100 miles from Krakow. Additionally, they set us up with the guide who was now leading us deep into the woods on what increasingly seemed like a dubious quest.

After what seemed like an eternity tromping through the forest, we suddenly came to a small clearing that was filled with gravestones. This ancient cemetery was completely overgrown with trees and bushes, and many of the tombstones had been knocked over but were still legible. After much hunting around, we managed to find a cluster of stones engraved with the names of some of our ancestors. Our attention was immediately riveted on one stone with the surname Kremsdorf, which had the correct dates and other details to be my great-great-grandfather's. Ellen, Judy, and I stood over our great-great-grandfather's gravestone and took a moment to pay our respects. Even though none of us had been to Poland before, it felt like we had truly returned to our roots.

◆

In New York City, my family's roots run deep. I was born and raised in the Bronx, and childhood memories come flooding back whenever I visit. After I won the Nobel Prize, I was invited back to New York for several events that ranked amongst the most moving experiences of my life.

One of these events was having my name engraved on the Nobel Monument. In September 2013, about a year after my Nobel Prize was announced, my family and I were invited to attend a grand ceremony in Theodore Roosevelt Park. This park is the location of the Nobel Monument, a huge bronze obelisk engraved with the names of all American Nobel Laureates. The location is especially significant to me, as Theodore Roosevelt Park borders on the Museum of Natural History, which was one of my favorite haunts as a child. I spent many afternoons with my father in the Museum of Natural History, fueling my passion for science.

The Nobel Monument is the sole monument in New York City that contains the names of living people. There's a city ordinance in New York stipulating that only the names of deceased individuals can be featured on monuments, but the Nobel Monument was granted special status as the lone exception to this law. At the ceremony, I got goosebumps as the giant cloth over the obelisk was removed and the new engravings were unveiled. It was simultaneously exciting, inspiring, and humbling to see my name up there with Theodore Roosevelt, Albert Einstein, John Steinbeck, and the many other legends.

The experience was even more special because I was joined by several dozen members of my extended family. When I learned I was invited to the ceremony, Lynn and I mentioned it to a few of my cousins who still live in and around New York City, and they spread the word to other family members. Soon, the event became a huge family reunion, with dozens of family members announcing they would attend. Lynn and I arranged for dinner afterward at an excellent Italian restaurant close to the park. We invited all of my relatives, including a number of younger cousins whom I had not previously met. A few of my other cousins put together beautiful displays of family photos through the years. The Associated Kremsdorf Descendants ("AKD's"; my father's side of the family) were well-represented, which was wonderful as I hadn't seen many of them since our regular gatherings during my childhood. My mother's side of the family was represented as well.

At one point in the evening, I meditated on the fact that almost everyone in the room was descended from ancestors who had fled terror, with many more who were not there because of the branches of my family that didn't make it out of Europe. This tragic history of my family somehow made the lives of the current generation seem all the sweeter. Like many descendants of refugees from the Holocaust and various pogroms, my cousins have all led rich lives, filled to the brim with family, love, and achievements. I'm no psychiatrist, but this incredible passion for living could be construed as an attempt to redeem the suffering of our ancestors, to show that we're not wasting the chance we've been given. The schmoozing and celebrating after the Nobel Monument ceremony continued unabated for many hours, and I left the party feeling elated to have reconnected with so many wonderful relatives.

A year later, I was invited back to New York for another special ceremony, this time at my alma mater Bronx Science. I had never been invited back to Bronx Science until I won the Nobel Prize; apparently, that's the level of achievement expected of the school's alumni in order to receive such an invitation. It is true that Bronx Science has produced more Nobel Laureates than any other secondary school in the world.

When I won the Nobel Prize in 2012, I was the eighth graduate of Bronx Science to win the prize. If Bronx Science was its own country, it would rank twenty-third in terms of total Nobel Prizes won, tied with Spain and ahead of Ireland, Finland, and more than 150 other nations. Most high schools have display cases exhibiting their sports trophies; Bronx Science has a display case in the main lobby showcasing the school's Nobel Laureates.

A special assembly was held in my honor, and the energy was unbelievable. I took a bunch of selfies with the students and also signed a ton of autographs. Amazingly, George Yancopoulos was on hand to introduce me before I spoke. George is the chief scientific officer of Regeneron Pharmaceuticals and a billionaire from all the successful drugs his company has developed. Like me, he's an alum of both Bronx Science and Columbia, and I was honored that he would show up to be my opening act.

After the assembly, I met with the current principal, Jean Donahue. She and her staff dug out some of my old documents from sixty years earlier. They had a piece of paper showing I scored 100 on the New York Regents Exam in math for three years in a row, an accomplishment that is still a point of pride for me, and they also had a full transcript with all my grades. They even had my application to Bronx Science, which I must've written when I was twelve years old. One of the questions was, *"What is your bedtime?"* and I had answered *"10:30 pm"*, which cracked me up because 10:30 P.M. was still my bedtime sixty years later. I guess some things never change.

At one point while walking around the school, I was approached by a wizened old woman with a devious smile.

"Do you know who I am?" she asked. I confessed that I couldn't recall, so she continued, "My name is Ms. Engel, and I was your tenth grade math teacher."

"Well, you obviously did a helluva job," I deadpanned. "The principal just showed me my New York Regents exams and I scored 100 on all of them!" Ms. Engel told me that she had retired long ago but was excited to return to the school for my ceremony. We shared a lot of laughs, and catching up with her was a highlight of the trip.

Another highlight of my visit was having the chance to spend time with several of my classmates, including Mike and Barbara Bertin, Bob Kurtz, June Golden, and Harriet Cohen Geller. All of these friends have worked with me over the years to help organize the Gene Frankel Science Essay contest. As mentioned in an earlier chapter, my best friend Gene Frankel demonstrated an unusual passion for the history of science as a high school student. He ended up living out his dream and becoming a highly respected science historian. Tragically, he died from cancer in his early forties. At the time of his death, I worked with a group of my classmates to establish a scholarship fund in Gene's honor, with the awards given to Bronx Science students who write outstanding essays on important deceased scientists. My classmates and I have served for many years on the committee that reviews the essays for the Frankel scholarships, and reviewing these essays each year reminds me of Gene and is immensely satisfying. It also keeps me in touch with these friends from a different era of my life some sixty years ago. However, in organizing this essay contest each year, my classmates and I mainly communicate via e-mail, so it was wonderful during my return to Bronx Science to have a whole day to spend time with them in person, remembering departed friends like Gene and reminiscing about the old days.

◆

During my visit to the Bronx, I naturally spent some time thinking about my parents. Given my family history, such thoughts often morph into meditations about my own mortality. My father had his first heart attack at fifty, then had a string of additional heart attacks prior to his premature death. My mother also had her first heart attack in her fifties. Two of my four grandparents died at quite young ages. Thus, I have long known that genetics is not on my side.

As I write these words, I am seventy-six years of age. Heart disease has stalked me all my life, but somehow I've managed to survive and even thrive. If I dropped dead tomorrow, nobody would say that I died young. I've lived long enough to see all of my children grow up, get married, and lead fascinating lives. I've had the pleasure of getting to know my six grandchildren, who currently range in age from four to twenty-four. I've also lived long enough to reach the most contented time of my professional and personal life. Yes, I enjoyed being the young hotshot back in the early days. Now, though, I get to be the grand old man of the field, which is even better.

When I returned to Duke after my visit to Bronx Science, I reflected on how North Carolina has truly become my home. I've been there now for more than forty-five years. Poland is my ancestral homeland and New York City is the place where I grew up, but North Carolina is where my roots lay now. After my travels, I was excited to get back in town and tell my friends about my adventures in my old stomping grounds. I also felt charged up to get back in the lab and talk with my students and postdocs about their most recent findings. After all, there are always new things to discover. My heart raced as I thought about some of the current directions we were exploring. A slew of exciting studies had been in progress when I left, and I was eager to see the latest data and talk with my trainees about their newest stories.

NOTES

1. Matters of the Heart

1. This was a cardiac catheterization procedure known as a coronary angiography. In this procedure, a catheter is inserted into an artery in the thigh and threaded up to the heart in order to inject a dye. In my case, I didn't even need the dye to see that there was a major problem. Atherosclerotic plaques are rich in calcium, which lights up when imaged in this type of procedure. What I saw on the screen was the signal from the huge calcium deposits that had built up around the atherosclerotic plaques in my coronary arteries.

2. Young Man in a Hurry

1. The use of a single standardized test score to determine admission to Bronx Science has continued for the past six decades. However, this practice has become highly controversial as it does not result in classes that are ethnically diverse and moreover doesn't capture the full measure of students' potential.

2. Steve Rudolph obtained a Ph.D. in chemistry from Yale and pursued postdoctoral research in the areas of chemistry and chemical biology. However,

in his thirties he had a change of heart and decided that what he really wanted was to go into medicine. He ended his research, attended medical school, and became a practicing cardiologist and pillar of his community.

When Steve and I were best friends at Bronx Science, my goal in life was to become a physician and Steve's dream was to go into research. As it turned out, I focused my career on research and Steve became a beloved physician. Somehow, we lived out each other's dream.

3. The Mysteries of Medicine

1. A number of my classmates from medical school went on to illustrious careers. The two classmates specifically mentioned in this chapter are cases in point. Harold Varmus won a Nobel Prize in 1989 for the discovery of oncogenes, and then later became the director of the National Institutes of Health. Meanwhile, Robin Cook became a best-selling writer of medical thrillers such as *Coma*, *Brain*, and *Outbreak*.

2. Arna wanted to name our first son David after her deceased father. Since Arna selected the baby's first name, she asked me to pick the middle name. I chose Ian, mainly because I was a huge fan of the writer Ian Fleming and his best-selling books about the secret agent James Bond. So, yes, I named my firstborn son after my favorite spy novelist. I was barely out of my teens at the time, and this seemed to me a perfectly reasonable way to name a child.

4. "Who's in the house tonight?"

1. Sam Thier went on to a very distinguished career in medicine. He was named chair of Medicine at Yale University at a very young age, and then some years later became president of Brandeis University. Later in his career, he returned to Harvard as president of Partners HealthCare. Thier's counterpart in the chief resident swap, Bill Lovejoy, spent his entire career at Columbia as a prominent cardiologist.

2. The *Diagnostic and Statistical Manual of Mental Disorders* (DSM) is the bible of psychiatric diagnosis. The DSM is updated every few years to

include newly described conditions. Bulimia nervosa did not appear in the DSM until 1987, which is almost twenty years after I treated the famous actress during my junior residency year at Columbia.

3. I did not keep in touch with this actress, but I heard that she completely stopped her bulimic behavior after her hospitalization. She went on to have a long and healthy life, winning a number of major awards for her stage and film career.

5. The Yellow Berets

1. A total of ten Yellow Berets went on to become Nobel laureates, which is impressive considering the relatively small size of the program. In addition to myself, the Yellow Berets who won Nobel Prizes were Michael Brown, Joseph Goldstein, J. Michael Bishop, Harold Varmus, Alfred Gilman, Stanley Prusiner, Ferid Murad, Richard Axel, and Harvey Alter. Beyond these ten, many dozens more Yellow Berets have been inducted into the National Academy of Sciences and received other major research accolades. Brown and Goldstein, who served together as Yellow Berets and then won a Nobel Prize together two decades later, wrote an excellent piece in 2012 exploring the potential reasons why so many Yellow Berets went on to have such stellar research careers:

J. L. Goldstein and M. S. Brown, "A golden era of Nobel laureates," *Science* 338, no. 6110 (November 2012): 1033–4.

A more detailed description of the lives and scientific careers of many of the Yellow Berets can be found in the outstanding book *Medal Winners: How the Vietnam War Launched Nobel Careers* by Raymond Greenberg.

2. Acromegaly is most often caused by benign tumors of the pituitary gland, known as pituitary adenomas, which cause the gland to release too much human growth hormone. If such excessive release happens during childhood, the result is gigantism, and the patient grows up to be unusually tall and muscular. In contrast, if the spike in growth hormone levels occurs after puberty or later, when the bones have already fused, the result

is an increase in the growth of certain features. For example, acromegalics who develop pituitary adenomas as adults typically have prominent jaws and large hands. The most common treatment for acromegaly is surgical removal of the pituitary adenoma.

3. Adrenocorticotropic hormone (ACTH) is secreted by the pituitary gland, often in response to stress, and acts on the adrenal gland to promote secretion of cortisol and other hormones. Given that the adrenal gland was known to respond to ACTH, Jesse and Ira postulated that adrenal tissue must contain a receptor that receives the ACTH signal. To label this hypothetical receptor, I first needed to label ACTH with a radioactive tag using a technique that Jesse had learned from his legendary mentor, the Nobel Laureate Rosalyn Yalow. Specifically, my project was focused on labeling ACTH with Iodine-125 (125I), then separating 125I-labled ACTH from the unlabeled hormone. I also needed to perform functional studies with 125I-ACTH to show that it was still biologically active, because the addition of a tag to the hormone might conceivably disrupt the ability of the hormone to activate its receptor. The ultimate goal was to use the 125I-ACTH to study binding of the hormone to its putative receptor. If binding could be achieved, then this binding assay could be used to measure the levels of ACTH in bodily fluids. At the time, there was no way to measure the levels of ACTH in the body, so this was an important goal.

4. The three papers published based on my work at the NIH were:

R. J. Lefkowitz, J. Roth, W. Pricer, and I. Pastan, "ACTH receptors in the adrenal: specific binding of ACTH-125I and its relation to adenyl cyclase," *Proceedings of the National Academy of Sciences USA* 65, no. 3 (March 1970): 745–52.

R. J. Lefkowitz, J. Roth, and I. Pastan, "Radioreceptor assay of adrenocorticotropic hormone: new approach to assay of polypeptide hormones in plasma," *Science* 170, no. 3968 (November 1970): 633–5.

R. J. Lefkowitz, J. Roth, and I. Pastan, "Effects of calcium on ACTH stimulation of the adrenal: separation of hormone binding from adenyl cyclase activation," *Nature* 228 (November 1970): 864–6.

6. Breaking the Rules at Mass General

1. Patients with acromegaly due to a pituitary tumor often exhibit pan-hypopituitarism, a general decrease in pituitary function. Such patients have low levels of ACTH and other hormones involved in the stress response, and thus their bodies do not respond well to stress, such as the stress of a surgery. Normally, ACTH triggers the release of cortisol from the adrenal gland to raise blood pressure and exert other effects in response to stress, but patients with pituitary tumors often lack the ACTH surge that is supposed to lead to the increased cortisol secretion. Thus, to compensate for the low cortisol levels, such patients can be given prednisone, a drug that mimics the action of cortisol.

2. There was some drama during the move, as we arrived at our new house on June 30, 1970, but had been unable to sign the loan papers. As a veteran of the Public Health Service, I was eligible for a VA loan with zero down payment. However, it turned out that I wasn't a veteran until the next day, July 1, when I was to be formally discharged from the Public Health Service. Fortunately, after talking on the phone to a dozen different people in a dozen different departments, I found a sympathetic government official who was willing to sign off on the loan even though I was technically not a veteran until the following day.

3. These binding studies revealed specific binding of 3H (tritium)–labeled noradrenaline that could be displaced by beta blockers such as propranolol. However, the eventual conclusion was that these binding sites did *not* actually represent the physiological beta-adrenergic receptor because: *i)* it took very high concentrations of beta blockers to displace the adrenaline binding, much higher than clinically relevant doses; and *ii)* the pharmacological profile of these binding sites did not match physiological beta receptors in other ways, for example in terms of the stereospecificity of ligand binding. To this day, it is still unclear what the 3H-noradrenaline in these assays was actually binding. Nonetheless, we published these findings as precursors of our ultimately successful attempts to characterize ligand binding to beta-adrenergic receptors:

R. J. Lefkowitz and E. Haber, "A fraction of the ventricular myocardium that has the specificity of the cardiac beta-adrenergic receptor," *Proceedings of the National Academy of Sciences USA* 68, no. 8 (August 1971): 1773–7.

R. J. Lefkowitz, E. Haber, and D. O'Hara, Identification of the cardiac beta-adrenergic receptor protein: solubilization and purification by affinity chromatography," *Proceedings of the National Academy of Sciences USA* 69, no. 10 (October 1972): 2828–32.

R. J. Lefkowitz, G. W. Sharp, and E. Haber, "Specific binding of beta-adrenergic catecholamines to a subcellular fraction from cardiac muscle," *Journal of Biological Chemistry* 248 (January 1973): 342–9.

4. Even though Silvio Cella had a rough season coaching Revere High School during my first year as the team physician, he eventually went on to a very distinguished coaching career and ended up being inducted into both the Massachusetts High School Coaches Hall of Fame and the National Football Federation Hall of Fame. He is the namesake of the Silvio Cella Family Foundation, which supports football player safety and also helps prepare student athletes for college, careers, and family: https://silvio cellafoundation.org.

7. "Duke? I never heard of it."

1. The two other groups competing with us to develop binding assays for labeling beta-adrenergic receptors were the Levitzki group at the Hebrew University in Jerusalem and the Aurbach group at the NIH. Levitzki and colleagues were studying the binding of radiolabeled propranolol to beta receptors, whereas the Aurbach group was studying the binding of radiolabeled hydroxybenzylpindolol. Our choice of alprenolol was based on the fact that it had a three-carbon aliphatic chain containing an unsaturated bond in a region remote from the core part of the molecule. We realized that New England Nuclear would be able to use the process of catalytic hydrogenation with tritium to insert two atoms of tritium across this double bond, thereby doubling the specific radioactivity and facilitating binding studies. Radiolabeled alprenolol is the only one of the three original radioligands

that remains in use today, almost a half-century later, as a tool for labeling beta receptors.

2. The key papers published in 1974–1975 describing our early binding assays with tritiated alprenolol were:

R. J. Lefkowitz, C. Mukherjee, M. Coverstone, and M. G. Caron, "Stereospecific (3H)(minus)-alprenolol binding sites, beta-adrenergic receptors and adenylate cyclase," *Biochemical and Biophysical Research Communications* 60, no. 2 (August 1974):703–9.

R. W. Alexander, L. T. Williams, and R. J. Lefkowitz, "Identification of cardiac beta-adrenergic receptors by (minus) [3H]alprenolol binding," *Proceedings of the National Academy of Sciences USA* 72, no. 4 (April 1975): 1564–8.

C. Mukherjee, M. G. Caron, M. Coverstone, and R. J. Lefkowitz, "Identification of adenylate cyclase-coupled beta-adrenergic receptors in frog erythrocytes with (minus)-[3-H] alprenolol," *Journal of Biological Chemistry* 250 no. 13 (July 1975): 4869–76.

R. W. Alexander, J. N. Davis, and R. J. Lefkowitz, "Direct identification and characterisation of beta-adrenergic receptors in rat brain." *Nature* 258 (December 1975): 437–40.

8. Travelin' Man

1. It is now well-known that Halcion does not induce sleepwalking per se, but rather induces anterograde amnesia. This means that patients taking Halcion may function normally for a number of hours, but then completely forget events that occurred while they were under the influence of the drug. In fact, recent research indicates that the main problem is that the drug actually blocks the formation of new memories. This side effect is particularly prominent in patients taking high doses of Halcion, but can be avoided if one sleeps until the medication has worn off. After my experience of profound anterograde amnesia on the flight from London after a high dose of Halcion, I would still take Halcion on occasion to sleep on overnight flights, but only at much lower doses,

which I found gave me the sleep-inducing benefits without the amnestic side effects.

10. The Howard Hughes Medical Institute

1. Despite the Mafia-like manner in which HHMI investigators were appointed in 1976, the capos who made the selections still managed to do an impressive job. In addition to myself, the class of '76 was comprised of David Garbers, John Glomset, Joel Habener, Y. W. Kan, Richard Palmiter, Stanley Prusiner, David Valle, and Savio Woo. All nine of these investigators had distinguished careers, with six of us being selected to the US National Academy of Sciences and two of us (Prusiner and myself) winning the Nobel Prize. Additionally, Palmiter and I are the two longest-tenured investigators in the history of HHMI, having each been funded for forty-three years and counting, as of this writing. The current system by which HHMI appointments are made is undeniably more fair and meritocratic, but nonetheless it should be recognized that the capos in 1976 did a pretty decent job of identifying future stars.

2. Fredrickson ended up serving as HHMI director for only a few years before resigning in scandal. When HHMI moved their headquarters from Florida to Maryland, Fredrickson's wife ("Madame") was put in charge of decorating the new headquarters. Madame had a taste for luxurious furnishings and spent an enormous sum on the new headquarters' interior design. It was rumored that this spending did not sit well with the HHMI board, which asked Fredrickson to resign. Fredrickson was replaced by Purnell Choppin, who ushered in a new era of highly professional management at HHMI and also oversaw a tremendous diversification in the ranks of HHMI investigators.

3. I had seen this same postdoc give a presentation the year before at a regional cardiovascular conference. During his talk, his voice had slowed like an old-fashioned record player running out of battery power until he eventually face-planted on the stage. Given the evidence that this postdoc was prone to fainting under pressure, it is unclear to me why

his mentor took the risk of putting him in front of the Howard Hughes review committee.

11. Two Thousand Frogs a Week

1. The article containing the skeptical quote from Ahlquist about the existence of receptors as physical entities is:

R. P. Ahlquist, "Adrenergic receptors: a personal and practical view," *Perspectives in. Biology and Medicine* 17, no. 1 (Autumn 1973): 119–22.

2. Prior to purification, we needed to find a way to remove the receptors from the cell membranes in which they resided. This would require a process known as solubilization, which means getting the receptors out of the cell membrane and into solution. In the mid-1970s, Marc Caron in my lab tried twenty different detergents to see if he could extract the beta-adrenergic receptors from cell membranes (i.e., solubilize them) in a functional form, that is to say, in a manner that allowed them to retain their ability to bind beta blockers. For nineteen of the twenty detergents he tried, Marc found no evidence of functional solubilized receptors, which was very disappointing. However, one of the detergents, a plant extract known as digitonin, resulted in clear evidence of solubilization of receptors that still bound to beta blockers and also bound to adrenaline.

3. Our primary purification approach was to link the beta blocker alprenolol to tiny sepharose beads. In our binding studies, we were using radiolabeled alprenolol as a tag that bound to beta receptors in order to detect them. In the purification studies, we would use alprenolol more like a fishing hook, with the sepharose beads being like tiny fishing rods that we would use to fish out beta receptors from solubilized tissue extracts, followed by elution from the sepharose beads using a competing solution of free alprenolol. After purification on the alprenolol sepharose column, we would then perform additional purification steps, often with high-performance liquid chromatography (HPLC) columns that Rob Shorr had commandeered from sales reps.

During these extended purification efforts, we burned through enormous quantities of digitonin. Moreover, we kept finding that not all digitonin samples were created equal. Digitonin is an extract derived from the digitalis plant, and in our hands some digitonin samples were much better than others in terms of solubilizing the receptors. For this reason, whenever we found a sample of digitonin that worked, we would contact the company and tell them we wanted to purchase the whole lot. One time, we spent $50,000 to buy the entire lot of a particularly good batch of digitonin. Fortunately, the Howard Hughes Medical Institute had increased our lab's funding that year, so we were able to afford such extravagances. Digitonin was absolutely essential to our experiments, so it was literally worth its weight in gold to us.

As we began to publish papers about our purification successes, people began writing to us asking for digitonin. They told us they'd tried to order it from the vendor, who told them that the Lefkowitz lab at Duke had purchased every last drop of digitonin they had in stock. Purifying digitonin from the digitalis plant was a laborious process and it took the vendors months to replenish their stocks, so we had unintentionally cornered the market on digitonin and caused a worldwide shortage. We did our best to share some of our digitonin supply with labs who wrote to us, but of course we couldn't share a large amount because we needed such massive quantities for our ongoing purification efforts.

4. Key papers reporting our beta-adrenergic receptor purification efforts from this era include:

M. G. Caron and R. J. Lefkowitz, "Solubilization and characterization of the beta-adrenergic receptor binding sites of frog erythrocytes" *Journal of Biological Chemistry* 251, no. 8 (April 1976): 2374–84.

M. G. Caron, Y. Srinivasan, J. Pitha, K. Kociolek, and R. J. Lefkowitz, "Affinity chromatography of the beta-adrenergic receptor," *Journal of Biological Chemistry* 254, no. 8 (April 1979): 2923–7.

R. G. Shorr, R. J. Lefkowitz, and M. G. Caron, "Purification of the beta-adrenergic receptor. Identification of the hormone binding subunit," *Journal of Biological Chemistry* 256, no. 11 (June 1981): 5820–6.

J. L. Benovic, R. G. Shorr, M. G. Caron, and R. J. Lefkowitz, "The mammalian beta 2-adrenergic receptor: purification and characterization," *Biochemistry* 23, no. 20 (September 1984): 4510–8.

5. A surprising problem we encountered in our reconstitution efforts was that it was difficult to find cells that didn't have any beta receptors. Beta-adrenergic receptors are found in almost all cell types in the body, so we screened numerous different cell types but were unable to find one that didn't already contain beta receptors. Then, we remembered our earlier screens of various amphibians and recalled that the red blood cells from the African clawed toad had shocked us because they contained *no* beta receptors at all. This cell type turned out to be the perfect choice for the reconstitution experiments, and Rick Cerione worked with several other people in the lab to demonstrate that addition of our purified beta receptors to the toad red blood cells was sufficient to confer responses to adrenaline and other adrenergic ligands.

The technical approach by which we accomplished this feat was to fuse the lipid vesicles containing the isolated beta-adrenergic receptor protein with the toad erythrocytes using polyethylene glycol as the fusogenic agent. As the artificial lipid membranes fused with the natural membranes of the red blood cells, the precious receptor cargo was inserted into the red blood cell membrane and was able to link up with the other components of the system that were naturally expressed there, including the G proteins and the adenylyl cyclase enzyme.

6. Key papers reporting our beta-adrenergic receptor reconstitution studies include:

R. A. Cerione, B. Strulovici, J. L. Benovic, C. D. Strader, M. G. Caron, and R. J. Lefkowitz, "Reconstitution of beta-adrenergic receptors in lipid vesicles: affinity chromatography-purified receptors confer catecholamine responsiveness on a heterologous adenylate cyclase system," *Proceedings of the National Academy of Sciences USA* 80, no. 16 (August 1983): 4899–903.

R. A. Cerione, B. Strulovici, J. L. Benovic, R. J. Lefkowitz, and M. G. Caron, "Pure beta-adrenergic receptor: the single polypeptide confers catecholamine responsiveness to adenylate cyclase," *Nature* 306 (December 1983): 562–6.

R. A. Cerione, D. R. Sibley, J. Codina, J. L. Benovic, J. Winslow, E. J. Neer, L. Birnbaumer, M. G. Caron, and R. J. Lefkowitz, "Reconstitution of a hormone-sensitive adenylate cyclase system. The pure beta-adrenergic receptor and guanine nucleotide regulatory protein confer hormone responsiveness on the resolved catalytic unit," *Journal of Biological Chemistry* 259, no. 16 (August 1984): 9979–82.

7. The most important model that André developed was known as the "ternary complex model." The word "ternary" refers to the three interacting components involved in ligand binding: the ligand, the receptor, and the G protein. This model holds that agonist binding promotes receptor coupling to G proteins. Reciprocally, receptor interactions with G proteins increase receptor affinity for agonists. These changes in affinity are not observed with antagonists, which explained why our binding curves for agonists and antagonists looked so different. This model also explained why our binding curves for agonists (but not antagonists) were influenced by addition of guanosine triphosphate (GTP), as the GTP modulated the G proteins to affect agonist binding.

A. De Léan, J. M. Stadel, and R. J. Lefkowitz, "A ternary complex model explains the agonist-specific binding properties of the adenylate cyclase-coupled beta-adrenergic receptor," *Journal of Biological Chemistry* 255, no. 15 (August 1980): 7108–17.

R. S. Kent, A. De Léan, and R. J. Lefkowitz, "A quantitative analysis of beta-adrenergic receptor interactions: resolution of high and low affinity states of the receptor by computer modeling of ligand binding data," *Molecular Pharmacology* 17, no. 1 (January 1980): 14–23.

In addition to the ternary complex model, André and Ernst also developed models for analyzing binding data for tissues expressing multiple subtypes of receptor. Many tissues in the body express multiple subtypes of closely related receptors: for example, the heart expresses both beta-1 and beta-2 adrenergic receptors, which bind to many of the same ligands.

Binding data derived from such tissues can be quite complex and require complicated computer-fitting techniques. The models developed by André and Ernst were amongst the first models of this type to analyze such binding data involving multiple receptor subtypes.

E. Bürgisser, A. A. Hancock, R. J. Lefkowitz, and A. De Léan, "Anomalous equilibrium binding properties of high-affinity racemic radioligands," *Molecular Pharmacology* 19, no. 2 (March 1981): 205–16.

A. De Léan, A. A. Hancock, and R. J. Lefkowitz, "Validation and statistical analysis of a computer modeling method for quantitative analysis of radioligand binding data for mixtures of pharmacological receptor subtypes," *Molecular Pharmacology* 21, no. 1 (January 1982): 5–16.

E. Bürgisser, A. De Léan, and R. J. Lefkowitz, "Reciprocal modulation of agonist and antagonist binding to muscarinic cholinergic receptor by guanine nucleotide," *Proceedings of the National Academy of Sciences USA* 79, no. 6 (March 1982): 1732–6.

When André left my lab, he took a faculty position at the University of Montreal, where he ultimately served as Chair of Pharmacology for more than a decade. André was never one to take the expected route, though, and true to form he ended up retiring early from his career in biological research to pursue studies in astronomy.

8. Key papers reporting our purification efforts focused on alpha adrenergic receptors include:

J. W. Regan, N. Barden, R. J. Lefkowitz, M. G. Caron, R. M. DeMarinis, A. J. Krog, K. G. Holden, W. D. Matthews, and J. B. Hieble, "Affinity chromatography of human platelet alpha 2-adrenergic receptors," *Proceedings of the National Academy of Sciences USA* 79, no. 23 (December 1982): 7223–7.

L. M. Leeb-Lundberg, K. E. Dickinson, S. L. Heald, J. E. Wikberg, P. O. Hagen, J. F. DeBernardis, M. Winn, D. L. Arendsen, R. J. Lefkowitz, and M. G. Caron, "Photoaffinity labeling of mammalian alpha 1-adrenergic receptors. Identification of the ligand binding subunit with a high affinity radioiodinated probe," *Journal of Biological Chemistry* 259, no. 4 (February 1984): 2579–87.

J. W. Regan, H. Nakata, R. M. DeMarinis, M. G. Caron, and R. J. Lefkowitz, "Purification and characterization of the human platelet alpha 2-adrenergic receptor," *Journal of Biological Chemistry* 261, no. 8 (December 1986): 3894–900.

J. W. Lomasney, L. M. Leeb-Lundberg, S. Cotecchia, J. W. Regan, J. F. DeBernardis, M. G. Caron, and R. J. Lefkowitz, "Mammalian alpha 1-adrenergic receptor. Purification and characterization of the native receptor ligand binding subunit," *Journal of Biological Chemistry* 261, no. 17 (May 1986): 7710–6.

12. "Mystery Physician Saves Man's Life"

1. Mickey and Newman were each very productive during their one year in the lab, and then both went on to very successful careers. Mickey published three important papers about ligand binding to beta-adrenergic receptors, and on two of these papers he was the lead author. I wrote a reference letter to help Long John obtain a residency at my old stomping grounds at Mass General, and ultimately he became an accomplished physician practicing internal medicine in Hawaii, which is definitely not a bad place to spend a career.

Needle Newman published a single lead-author paper based on his year in my lab, but it was a very high-profile paper in the *Journal of Clinical Investigation*. Newman later went on to become a distinguished pediatric surgeon at George Washington University School of Medicine and eventually president and CEO of Children's National Health System. He published a terrific book in 2017 entitled *Healing Children: A Surgeon's Stories from the Frontiers of Pediatric Medicine*. The citations for the papers from Mickey and Newman are:

J. Mickey, R. Tate, and R. J. Lefkowitz, "Subsensitivity of adenylate cyclase and decreased beta-adrenergic receptor binding after chronic exposure to (minus)-isoproterenol in vitro," *Journal of Biological Chemistry* 250 (July 1975): 5727–9.

J. V. Mickey, R. Tate, D. Mullikin, and R. J. Lefkowitz, "Regulation of adenylate cyclase-coupled beta adrenergic receptor binding sites by beta adrenergic catecholamines in vitro," *Molecular Pharmacology* 12, no. 3 (May 1976): 409–19.

R. J. Lefkowitz, C. Mukherjee, L. E. Limbird, M. G. Caron, L. T. Williams, R. W. Alexander, J. V. Mickey, and R. Tate, "Regulation of adenylate cyclase coupled beta-adrenergic receptors," *Recent Progress in Hormone Research* 32 (1976): 597–632.

K. D. Newman, L. T. Williams, N. H. Bishopric, and R. J. Lefkowitz, "Identification of alpha-adrenergic receptors in human platelets by [3H] dihydroergocryptine binding," *The Journal of Clinical Investigation* 61, no. 2 (February 1978): 395–402.

13. The Quest for the Holy Grail

1. In the sole criticism that we received from the reviewers of our manuscript at *Nature*, one of the reviewers asked, *"Why are you not concerned that this is a pseudogene?"*

"Well," I joked in a meeting with my coauthors, "The reason why I'm not concerned is that I have never heard of a pseudogene!"

I soon learned that a pseudogene was a stretch of DNA that looks like a gene but is not actually expressed by cells. To address the reviewer's comment, we simply used the sequence that Brian had pulled out of the genomic library to design a new probe for the beta receptor gene, then demonstrated that this probe recognized clones from a cDNA library (e.g., a library containing only genes that are actually expressed in cells). We showed that this clone had the same sequence as our original genomic clone.

2. The reference for the paper describing the cloning of the beta-2 adrenergic receptor is:

R. A. Dixon, B. K. Kobilka, D. J. Strader, J. L. Benovic, H. G. Dohlman, T. Frielle, M. A. Bolanowski, C. D. Bennett, E. Rands, R. E. Diehl, R. A. Mumford, E. E. Slater, I. S. Sigal, M. G. Caron, R. J. Lefkowitz, and C. D. Strader, "Cloning of the gene and cDNA for

mammalian beta-adrenergic receptor and homology with rhodopsin," *Nature* 321 (May 1986): 75–79.

My only regret about this paper is that I felt the author list didn't give
Brian Kobilka the appropriate credit. The first and last author positions of
scientific papers are typically reserved for the authors who made the most
significant contributions to the work. As part of the deal that I struck with
Ed Scolnick at the beginning of our collaboration, Merck was entitled to
both the first and last author positions on any resultant manuscript. Thus,
Dixon became the first author and Strader the last author. Given how things
turned out, I always felt that the balance of contributions shifted significantly during the course of the collaboration, and therefore the Duke team
should've ended up with at least one (if not both) of the key author positions.
Not only did my lab at Duke provide the purified receptor that was the key
to the whole effort, but we also provided several key breakthroughs on the
molecular biology side, including the crucial development of the genomic
library that led to the true breakthrough in the project.

In my opinion, Brian was the MVP of the cloning effort and therefore
was deserving of a first authorship or at least "co-first authorship." This
practice of having multiple lead authors on scientific papers is relatively
common these days, but unfortunately was not yet in practice at the time.
My view of Brian's central role certainly doesn't take anything away from
Richard Dixon, who made important contributions to the project and also
served as Brian's molecular biology mentor, but Brian's hard work and
creative ideas were what truly put us over the top in the race against Ross
and Ullrich. Brian is a selfless person by nature, a total team player, so he
repeatedly insisted that his authorship position didn't matter to him at all.
In any case, I learned the lesson to never negotiate authorship positions
until a project is over and the actual contributions of everyone involved
can be fully evaluated.

3. Ross and Ullrich submitted their manuscript to *Science*, which along with
Nature is one of the top scientific journals in the world. However, after the
Science editors saw our paper come out in *Nature*, they declined to publish
the Ross and Ullrich paper, saying it was merely confirmatory. This is how

scientific publishing goes: novelty means everything, and if you're not the first to publish a given gene sequence or crystal structure or groundbreaking idea, then it can be difficult to publish your paper once somebody else beats you to the punch. The rejection from *Science* must have been particularly galling for Ross and Ullrich because the two receptor clones were in fact completely different subtypes from different species: our sequence was the beta-2 adrenergic receptor from hamster and theirs was a beta-1 receptor from turkey. Ross and Ullrich eventually published their work in *Proceedings of the National Academy of Sciences USA*. The publication date for their paper was September 1986, which was a full four months after our paper had come out in *Nature*. This made the race to clone the beta receptor gene look like a blowout, when in fact it had been a photo finish.

Y. Yarden, H. Rodriguez, S. K.-F. Wong, D. R. Brandt, D. C. May, J. Burnier, R. N. Harkins, E. Y. Chen, J. Ramachandran, A. Ullrich, and E. M. Ross, "The avian beta-adrenergic receptor: primary structure and membrane topology," *Proceedings of the National Academy of Sciences USA* 83, no. 18 (September 1986): 6795–9.

14. The Rosetta Stone

1. Two years earlier, when the rhodopsin sequence had been worked out in 1984, the only other sequence it looked like was that of bacteriorhodopsin, a light-sensitive proton pump found in archaebacteria. Thus, it was presumed that the seven-transmembrane structure must be characteristic of light-sensitive proteins. When we demonstrated that the beta-2 adrenergic receptor had a seven-transmembrane structure, it immediately suggested that this was not a signature of light-sensitive proteins but instead was a characteristic of G protein–coupled receptors.

In hindsight, there were obvious parallels between the beta-2 adrenergic receptor and rhodopsin that suggested they might be related. Both activated a GTP-binding protein (transducin in the case of rhodopsin, Gs in the case of the beta-2 receptor); both were known to regulate cyclic nucleotide levels (cyclic GMP in the case of rhodopsin, cyclic AMP for the beta receptor); and both were known to be solubilized in a functional form by digitonin.

NOTES

At the time, though, rhodopsin was not thought of as a receptor in any traditional sense, which is why nobody expected the beta-2 receptor and rhodopsin to be even remotely similar to each other and why the similarity in their sequences and domain architecture came as such a shock.

2. The references for the cloning of the beta-1 receptor, as well as the first alpha-1 receptor and first alpha-2 receptor, are:

T. Frielle, S. Collins, K. W. Daniel, M. G. Caron, R. J. Lefkowitz, and B. K. Kobilka, "Cloning of the cDNA for the human beta 1-adrenergic receptor," *Proceedings of the National Academy of Sciences USA* 84, no. 22 (November 1987): 7920–4.

B. K. Kobilka, H. Matsui, T. S. Kobilka, T. L. Yang-Feng, U. Francke, M. G. Caron, R. J. Lefkowitz, and J. W. Regan, "Cloning, sequencing, and expression of the gene coding for the human platelet alpha 2-adrenergic receptor," *Science* 238, no. 4827 (October 1987): 650–6.

S. Cotecchia, D. A. Schwinn, R. R. Randall, R. J. Lefkowitz, M. G. Caron, and B. K. Kobilka, "Molecular cloning and expression of the cDNA for the hamster alpha 1-adrenergic receptor," *Proceedings of the National Academy of Sciences USA* 85, no. 19 (October 1988): 7159–63.

3. The realization that there were actually multiple subtypes of alpha-1 and alpha-2 receptors was fascinating in terms of the basic biology and also exciting in terms of drug development. Given that alpha-1 and alpha-2 receptors were already important drug targets at the time (for treating high blood pressure, amongst other conditions), the existence of multiple subtypes of these receptors with distinct tissue distributions offered the possibility of developing drugs targeting alpha receptors with more tissue-specific actions and fewer side effects. The references for the identification of the gene sequences for the additional alpha receptor subtypes are:

J. W. Regan, T. S. Kobilka, T. L. Yang-Feng, M. G. Caron, R. J. Lefkowitz, and B. K. Kobilka, "Cloning and expression of a human kidney cDNA for an alpha 2-adrenergic receptor subtype," *Proceedings of the National Academy of Sciences USA* 85, no. 17 (September 1988): 6301–5.

286

D. A. Schwinn, J. W. Lomasney, W. Lorenz, P. J. Szklut, R. T. Fremeau Jr, T. L. Yang-Feng, M. G. Caron, R. J. Lefkowitz, and S. Cotecchia, "Molecular cloning and expression of the cDNA for a novel alpha 1-adrenergic receptor subtype," *Journal of Biological Chemistry* 265, no. 14 (May 1990): 8183–9.

J. W. Lomasney, W. Lorenz, L. F. Allen, K. King, J. W. Regan, T. L. Yang-Feng, M. G. Caron, and R. J. Lefkowitz, "Expansion of the alpha 2-adrenergic receptor family: cloning and characterization of a human alpha 2-adrenergic receptor subtype, the gene for which is located on chromosome 2," *Proceedings of the National Academy of Sciences USA* 87, no. 13 (July 1990): 5094–8.

J. W. Lomasney, S. Cotecchia, W. Lorenz, W. Y. Leung, D. A. Schwinn, T. L. Yang-Feng, M. Brownstein, R. J. Lefkowitz, and M. G. Caron, "Molecular cloning and expression of the cDNA for the alpha 1A-adrenergic receptor. The gene for which is located on human chromosome 5," *Journal of Biological Chemistry* 266, no. 10 (April 1991): 6365–9.

In follow-up studies, we also examined the distribution of the various alpha-1 receptor subtypes throughout the body. One of our most impactful papers in this area was spearheaded by a urology resident named David Price, who worked in my lab for a few years. David found that the prostate gland was enriched in one particular subtype of alpha-1 receptor, which was distinct from the subtype dominantly expressed in blood vessels. This information would prove to be important later in the decade as various drug companies developed subtype-specific alpha-1 receptor blockers (such as Flomax and Rapaflo) to treat men suffering from an enlarged prostate gland (a condition also known as "benign prostatic hyperplasia," or BPH). We did not make any money from the development of these drugs, but were happy to have contributed to the basic research that made their development possible. Our work in this area was published in the *Journal of Urology*, the only publication of my career in this journal:

D. T. Price, D. A. Schwinn, J. W. Lomasney, L. F. Allen, M. G. Caron, and R. J. Lefkowitz, "Identification, quantification, and localization of mRNA for three distinct alpha 1 adrenergic receptor subtypes in human prostate," *Journal of Urology* 150, no. 2 part 1 (August 1993): 546–51.

4. When we first identified the mystery sequence that was similar to the beta-2 receptor, it was named "G-21," as mentioned earlier. Even though we had no idea what this receptor was, we published it in *Nature* because it was a new concept: the first orphan receptor, a term indicating a receptor that is not yet paired with a ligand. Today, vast numbers of orphan receptors are known, and many labs around the world are focused on trying to match up these receptors with ligands that might activate them.

In the case of G-21, we discovered that the expressed receptor weakly bound to beta blockers such as radiolabeled alprenolol. However, this binding was not displaced by adrenaline or other adrenergic ligands, so we knew it was not an adrenergic receptor. Annick Fargin, a postdoc in the lab, found some papers showing that certain serotonin receptors could bind weakly to beta blockers, so she and John Raymond tested whether G-21 might be a serotonin receptor, and indeed it was (the so-called serotonin 5-HT1A receptor). We then published these findings in *Nature* again, which meant that we ended up publishing the discovery of this receptor twice in *Nature*: once as an orphan and once as the serotonin 5-HT1A receptor!

B. K. Kobilka, T. Frielle, S. Collins, T. Yang-Feng, T. S. Kobilka, U. Francke, R. J. Lefkowitz, and M. G. Caron, "An intronless gene encoding a potential member of the family of receptors coupled to guanine nucleotide regulatory proteins," *Nature* 329, no. 6134 (September 1987): 75–79.

A. Fargin, J. R. Raymond, M. J. Lohse, B. K. Kobilka, M. G. Caron, and R. J. Lefkowitz, "The genomic clone G-21 which resembles a beta-adrenergic receptor sequence encodes the 5-HT1A receptor," *Nature* 335, no. 6188 (September 1988): 358–60.

5. References for our studies demonstrating phosphorylation of the beta-2 adrenergic receptor, as well as the importance of this phosphorylation in mediating receptor desensitization, include:

J. M. Stadel, P. Nambi, R. G. Shorr, D. F. Sawyer, M. G. Caron, and R. J. Lefkowitz, "Catecholamine-induced desensitization of turkey erythrocyte adenylate cyclase is associated with phosphorylation of the beta-adrenergic receptor," *Proceedings of the National Academy of Sciences USA* 80, no. 11 (June 1983): 3173–7.

B. Strulovici, R. A. Cerione, B. F. Kilpatrick, M. G. Caron, and R. J. Lefkowitz, "Direct demonstration of impaired functionality of a purified desensitized beta-adrenergic receptor in a reconstituted system," *Science* 225, no. 4664 (August 1984): 837–40.

P. Nambi, J. R. Peters, D. R. Sibley, and R. J. Lefkowitz, "Desensitization of the turkey erythrocyte beta-adrenergic receptor in a cell-free system. Evidence that multiple protein kinases can phosphorylate and desensitize the receptor," *Journal of Biological Chemistry* 260 (February 1985): 2165–71.

D. R. Sibley, R. H. Strasser, J. L. Benovic, K. Daniel, and R. J. Lefkowitz, "Phosphorylation/dephosphorylation of the beta-adrenergic receptor regulates its functional coupling to adenylate cyclase and subcellular distribution," *Proceedings of the National Academy of Sciences USA* 83, no. 24 (December 1986): 9408–12.

M. Bouvier, W. P. Hausdorff, A. De Blasi, B. F. O'Dowd, B. K. Kobilka, M. G. Caron, and R. J. Lefkowitz, "Removal of phosphorylation sites from the beta 2-adrenergic receptor delays onset of agonist-promoted desensitization," *Nature* 333, no. 6171 (May 1988): 370–3.

6. After we figured out the sequence for the gene encoding the beta receptor and realized its similarity to rhodopsin, this provided further insight because rhodopsin was already known to be phosphorylated by an enzyme called "rhodopsin kinase." We intuited that the kinase Scoop Benovic had purified (which we called "BARK" for "beta adrenergic receptor kinase") must be related to rhodopsin kinase. Indeed, Scoop showed that rhodopsin kinase was capable of phosphorylating the beta receptor, and BARK in turn was capable of phosphorylating rhodopsin. Ultimately, we identified the gene sequences for both BARK and rhodopsin kinase and showed them to be the founding members of a new family of kinases that play central roles in mediating receptor desensitization. References for the purification and

cloning of BARK, as well as the demonstration of the functional and sequence similarity between BARK and rhodopsin kinase, are:

J. L. Benovic, R. H. Strasser, M. G. Caron, and R. J. Lefkowitz, "Beta-adrenergic receptor kinase: identification of a novel protein kinase that phosphorylates the agonist-occupied form of the receptor," *Proceedings of the National Academy of Sciences USA* 83, no. 9 (May 1986): 2797–801.

J. L. Benovic, F. Mayor Jr, R. L. Somers, M. G. Caron, and R. J. Lefkowitz, "Light-dependent phosphorylation of rhodopsin by beta-adrenergic receptor kinase," *Nature* 321 (June 1986): 869–72.

J. L. Benovic, A. DeBlasi, W. C. Stone, M. G. Caron, and R. J. Lefkowitz, "Beta-adrenergic receptor kinase: primary structure delineates a multi-gene family," *Science* 246, no. 4927 (October 1989): 235–40.

W. Lorenz, J. Inglese, K. Palczewski, J. J. Onorato, M. G. Caron, and R. J. Lefkowitz, "The receptor kinase family: primary structure of rhodopsin kinase reveals similarities to the beta-adrenergic receptor kinase," *Proceedings of the National Academy of Sciences USA* 88, no. 19 (October 1991): 8715–9.

In later years, a number of additional members of this family of kinases would be identified. The family now has seven members and is referred to as the G protein-coupled receptor kinases (GRK1-7), with rhodopsin kinase being renamed GRK1 and BARK being renamed GRK2 as the founding members of the family.

7. The references for the elucidation of the gene sequences for the beta-arrestins are:

M. J. Lohse, J. L. Benovic, J. Codina, M. G. Caron, and R. J. Lefkowitz, "Beta-arrestin: a protein that regulates beta-adrenergic receptor function," *Science* 248, no. 4962 (June 1990): 1547–50.

H. Attramadal, J. L. Arriza, C. Aoki, T. M. Dawson, J. Codina, M. M. Kwatra, S. H. Snyder, M. G. Caron, and R. J. Lefkowitz, "Beta-arrestin2, a novel member of the arrestin/beta-arrestin gene family," *Journal of Biological Chemistry* 267, no. 25 (September 1992): 17882–90.

15. How to Fix a Broken Heart

1. A coronary bypass is a procedure that restores blood flow to the heart by channeling blood around blocked or narrowed regions of coronary arteries. This is done by grafting blood vessels from noncardiac areas into the heart to divert blood flow around such blockages. In my case, I had a quadruple bypass, which means four grafts were performed: two mammary artery grafts and two saphenous vein grafts. For the mammary artery grafts, my mammary arteries were cut and then grafted to the nearby coronary arteries to circumvent blockages. In the case of the saphenous vein grafts, two pieces of saphenous vein were removed from my legs and then each was plugged into the aorta at one end and into a blocked coronary artery beyond the obstruction at the other in order to bypass the obstruction.

2. In further discussions with colleagues months later, I would learn that it's not unusual for multiple attempts to be required to restart the heart following a coronary bypass. Sometimes the heart resumes beating on its own, but if it doesn't, then a mild electric shock is delivered. The shock is intentionally set at a low level, so multiple attempts can sometimes be needed. Of course, it's one thing to understand the principles involved, and another thing entirely when it's your own heart that proves difficult to restart. When I learned that it took four attempts to get my heart going again, I got a case of the willies that could not be assuaged no matter how many of my colleagues told me it was perfectly normal. After all, this was *my* heart we were talking about!

17. "Well, it's not the Nobel Prize . . ."

1. After spearheading the cloning of the alpha-1B adrenergic receptor in my lab, Susanna Cotecchia became interested in identifying the region of the receptor controlling coupling to G proteins. Since our earlier studies on the beta-2 and alpha-2 adrenergic receptors had identified the third cytoplasmic loops of these receptors as important for G protein coupling, Susanna began making mutations to the third loop of the alpha-1B receptor to try to block coupling to G proteins. Surprisingly, though, Susanna ended

up finding mutations that actually *increased* receptor signaling rather than blocking it. Moreover, the increases in signaling that she observed were independent of the presence of adrenaline or other agonists. That is to say, the mutant receptors were "constitutively active." Subsequently, we figured out how to make similar activating mutations to the third cytoplasmic loop of the beta-2 receptor. The key references for this work are as follows:

S. Cotecchia, S. Exum, M. G. Caron, and R. J. Lefkowitz, "Regions of the alpha 1-adrenergic receptor involved in coupling to phosphatidylinositol hydrolysis and enhanced sensitivity of biological function," *Proceedings of the National Academy of Sciences USA* 87, no. 8 (April 1990): 2896–900.

L. F. Allen, R. J. Lefkowitz, M. G. Caron, and S. Cotecchia, "G-protein-coupled receptor genes as protooncogenes: constitutively activating mutation of the alpha 1B-adrenergic receptor enhances mitogenesis and tumorigenicity," *Proceedings of the National Academy of Sciences USA* 88, no. 24 (December 1991): 11354–8.

M. A. Kjelsberg, S. Cotecchia, J. Ostrowski, M. G. Caron, and R. J. Lefkowitz, "Constitutive activation of the alpha 1B-adrenergic receptor by all amino acid substitutions at a single site. Evidence for a region which constrains receptor activation," *Journal of Biological Chemistry* 267, no. 3 (January 1992): 1430–3.

P. Samama, S. Cotecchia, T. Costa, and R. J. Lefkowitz, "A mutation-induced activated state of the beta 2-adrenergic receptor. Extending the ternary complex model," *Journal of Biological Chemistry* 268, no. 7 (March 1993): 4625–36.

G. Pei, P. Samama, M. Lohse, M. Wang, J. Codina, and R. J. Lefkowitz, "A constitutively active mutant beta 2-adrenergic receptor is constitutively desensitized and phosphorylated," *Proceedings of the National Academy of Sciences USA* 91, no. 7 (March 1994): 2699–702.

The idea that receptor mutations could lead to ligand-independent constitutive receptor signaling was a novel concept in pharmacology at the time. At first, these activating mutations seemed to be just a laboratory curiosity. However, over the next two decades, many groups around the world identified human diseases (thyroid adenomas, precocious male puberty, certain types of night blindness, et cetera) caused by constitutively activating mutations to G protein–coupled receptors. In some cases, the disease-associated mutations were found to be identical to mutations that we had made in the lab while performing basic research on constitutive signaling by adrenergic receptors. Thus, our basic research in this area set the table for understanding these genetic diseases.

2. The key references for the transgenic studies spearheaded by Carmelo Milano are as follows:

C. A. Milano, L. F. Allen, H. A. Rockman, P. C. Dolber, T. R. McMinn, K. R. Chien, T. D. Johnson, R. A. Bond, and R. J. Lefkowitz, "Enhanced myocardial function in transgenic mice overexpressing the beta 2-adrenergic receptor," *Science* 264, no. 5158 (April 1994): 582–6.

C. A. Milano, P. C. Dolber, H. A. Rockman, R. A. Bond, M. E. Venable, L. F. Allen, and R. J. Lefkowitz, "Myocardial expression of a constitutively active alpha 1B-adrenergic receptor in transgenic mice induces cardiac hypertrophy," *Proceedings of the National Academy of Sciences USA* 91, no. 21 (October 1994): 10109–13.

P. Samama, R. A. Bond, H. A. Rockman, C. A. Milano, and R. J. Lefkowitz, "Ligand-induced overexpression of a constitutively active beta2-adrenergic receptor: pharmacological creation of a phenotype in transgenic mice." *Proceedings of the National Academy of Sciences USA* 94, no. 1 (January 1997): 137–41.

3. Wally Koch worked with Carmelo Milano and others to make the surprising discovery that expressing a small fragment of the beta-adrenergic receptor kinase (BARK) in cardiac tissue exerted protective effects against cardiac damage. Subsequent studies demonstrated that this effect was mainly due to inhibition of signaling by the G protein subunits known as beta and gamma, which normally bind to BARK in a manner that increases the enzyme's activity by helping to localize BARK to the plasma membrane where the receptors reside. Conversely, overexpression of the BARK fragment could block this effect of the beta and gamma subunits. For

the next twenty-five years after the first report of this phenomenon, Wally continued following up these observations as an independent investigator, publishing paper after paper about transgenic and gene therapy approaches aimed at inhibiting beta and gamma subunits to protect the heart. The key references for the initial studies in this area that were made in my lab are:

W. J. Koch, B. E. Hawes, J. Inglese, L. M. Luttrell, and R. J. Lefkowitz, "Cellular expression of the carboxyl terminus of a G protein-coupled receptor kinase attenuates G beta gamma-mediated signaling," *Journal of Biological Chemistry* 269, no. 8 (February 1994): 6193–7.

W. J. Koch, H. A. Rockman, P. Samama, R. A. Hamilton, R. A. Bond, C. A. Milano, and R. J. Lefkowitz, "Cardiac function in mice overexpressing the beta-adrenergic receptor kinase or a beta ARK inhibitor," *Science* 268, no. 5215 (June 1995): 1350–3.

S. A. Akhter, C. A. Skaer, A. P. Kypson, P. H. McDonald, K. C. Peppel, D. D. Glower, R. J. Lefkowitz, and W. J. Koch. "Restoration of beta-adrenergic signaling in failing cardiac ventricular myocytes via adenoviral-mediated gene transfer," *Proceedings of the National Academy of Sciences USA* 94, no. 22 (October 1997): 12100–5.

18. *Jeopardy!*

1. The reference for the initial report from the Belgian group about sperm odorant receptors is:

M. Parmentier, F.Libert, S. Schurmans, S. Schiffmann, A. Lefort, D. Eggerickx, C. Ledent, C. Mollereau, C. Gérard, J. Perret, A. Grootegoed, and G. Vassart, "Expression of members of the putative olfactory receptor gene family in mammalian germ cells," *Nature* 355 (January 1992): 453–5.

2. The reference for my lab's article about mediation of stress responses by beta-2 adrenergic receptors is:

M. R. Hara, J. J. Kovacs, E. J. Whalen, S. Rajagopal, R. T. Strachan, W. Grant, A. J. Towers, B. Williams, C. M. Lam, K. Xiao, S. K. Shenoy,

S. G. Gregory, S. Ahn, D. R. Duckett, and R. J. Lefkowitz, "A stress response pathway regulates DNA damage through β2-adrenoreceptors and β-arrestin-1," *Nature* 477, no. 7364 (August 2011): 349–53.

3. The text for my ASCI presidential address can be found in the following reference:

R. J. Lefkowitz, "The spirit of science," *The Journal of Clinical Investigation* 82, no. 2 (August 1988): 375–8.

4. The text for my AAP presidential address can be found in the following reference:

R. J. Lefkowitz, "2001: An AAP (Association of American Physicians) odyssey," *The Journal of Clinical Investigation* 108, no. 7 (October 2001): s9–s13.

20. The Death Project

1. Some of the key papers reporting my lab's studies on proteins that differentially interact with beta-1 versus beta-2 adrenergic receptors are:

R. A. Hall, R. T. Premont, C. W. Chow, J. T. Blitzer, J. A. Pitcher, A. Claing, R. H. Stoffel, L. S. Barak, S. Shenolikar, E. J. Weinman, S. Grinstein, and R. J. Lefkowitz, "The beta-2-adrenergic receptor interacts with the Na+/H+-exchanger regulatory factor to control Na+/H+ exchange," *Nature* 392, no. 6676 (April 1998): 626–30.

Y. Tang, L. A. Hu, W. E. Miller, N. Ringstad, R. A. Hall, J. A. Pitcher, P. DeCamilli, and R. J. Lefkowitz, "Identification of the endophilins (SH3p4/p8/p13) as novel binding partners for the beta-1-adrenergic receptor," *Proceedings of the National Academy of Sciences USA* 96, no. 22 (October 1999): 12559–64.

L. A. Hu, Y. Tang, W. E. Miller, M. Cong, A. G. Lau, R. J. Lefkowitz, and R. A. Hall, "Beta-1-adrenergic receptor association with PSD-95: inhibition of receptor internalization and facilitation of beta-1-adrenergic receptor interaction with N-methyl-D-aspartate receptors," *Journal of Biological Chemistry* 275, no. 49 (December 2000): 38659–66.

M. Cong, S. J. Perry, L. A. Hu, P. I. Hanson, A. Claing, and R. J. Lefkowitz, "Binding of the beta-2 adrenergic receptor to N-ethylmaleimide-sensitive factor regulates receptor recycling," *Journal of Biological Chemistry* 276, no. 48 (November 2001): 45145–52.

2. The paper from Marc Caron's lab that first reported the role of beta-arrestins in mediating agonist-promoted receptor internalization is:

S. S. Ferguson, W. R. Downey III, A. M. Colapietro, L. S. Barak, L. Ménard, and M. G. Caron, "Role of beta-arrestin in mediating agonist-promoted G protein-coupled receptor internalization," *Science* 271, no. 5247 (January 1996): 363–6.

3. The paper from my lab first proposing a role for G protein–coupled receptor internalization in mediating certain aspects of receptor signaling is:

Y. Daaka, L. M. Luttrell, S. Ahn, G. J. Della Rocca, S. S. Ferguson, M. G. Caron, and R. J. Lefkowitz, "Essential role for G protein–coupled receptor endocytosis in the activation of mitogen-activated protein kinase," *Journal of Biological Chemistry* 273, no. 2 (January 1998): 685–8.

4. Some of my lab's early papers on beta-arrestin-mediated signaling by G protein–coupled receptors are:

L. M. Luttrell, S. S. Ferguson, Y. Daaka, W. E. Miller, S. Maudsley, G. J. Della Rocca, F. Lin, H. Kawakatsu, K. Owada, D. K. Luttrell, M. G. Caron, and R. J. Lefkowitz, "Beta-arrestin-dependent formation of beta2 adrenergic receptor-Src protein kinase complexes," *Science* 283, no. 5402 (January 1999): 655–61.

P. H. McDonald, C. W. Chow, W. E. Miller, S. A. Laporte, M. E. Field, F. T. Lin, R. J. Davis, and R. J. Lefkowitz, "Beta-arrestin 2: a receptor-regulated MAPK scaffold for the activation of JNK3," *Science* 290, no. 5496 (November 2000): 1574–7.

L. M. Luttrell, F. L. Roudabush, E. W. Choy, W. E. Miller, M. E. Field, K. L. Pierce, and R. J. Lefkowitz, "Activation and targeting of extracellular signal-regulated kinases by beta-arrestin scaffolds," *Proceedings of the National Academy of Sciences USA* 98, no. 5 (February 2001): 2449–54.

5. A comprehensive review article about the history of research on biased signaling by G protein–coupled receptors (a phenomenon also known as "functional selectivity") was published in 2007, and the reference is:

J. D. Urban, W. P. Clarke, M. von Zastrow, D. E. Nichols, B. Kobilka, H. Weinstein, J. A. Javitch, B. L. Roth, A. Christopoulos, P. M. Sexton, K. J. Miller, M. Spedding, and R. B. Mailman, "Functional selectivity and classical concepts of quantitative pharmacology," *The Journal of Pharmacology and Experimental Therapeutics* 320, no. 1 (January 2007): 1–13.

A later review article that focuses more specifically on biased signaling due to differential activation of G protein- vs. beta-arrestin-mediated is:

E. Reiter, S. Ahn, A. K. Shukla, and R. J. Lefkowitz, "Molecular mechanism of beta-arrestin-biased agonism at seven-transmembrane receptors," *Annual Review of Pharmacology and Toxicology* 52 (February 2012): 179–97.

6. Some of my lab's key studies on biased signaling by beta-adrenergic and angiotensin receptors are reported in the following papers:

H. Wei, S. Ahn, S. K. Shenoy, S. S. Karnik, L. Hunyady, L. M. Luttrell, and R. J. Lefkowitz, "Independent beta-arrestin 2 and G protein-mediated pathways for angiotensin II activation of extracellular signal-regulated kinases 1 and 2," *Proceedings of the National Academy of Sciences USA* 100, no. 19 (September 2003): 10782–7.
S. Ahn, S. K. Shenoy, H. Wei, and R. J. Lefkowitz, "Differential kinetic and spatial patterns of beta-arrestin and G protein-mediated ERK activation by the angiotensin II receptor," *Journal of Biological Chemistry* 279, no. 34 (August 2004): 35518–25.

K. Rajagopal, E. J. Whalen, J. D. Violin, J. A. Stiber, P. B. Rosenberg, R. T. Premont, T. M. Coffman, H. A. Rockman, and R. J. Lefkowitz, "Beta-arrestin2-mediated inotropic effects of the angiotensin II type 1A receptor in isolated cardiac myocytes," *Proceedings of the National Academy of Sciences USA* 103, no. 44 (October 2006): 16284–9.

J. W. Wisler, S. M. DeWire, E. J. Whalen, J. D. Violin, M. T. Drake, S. Ahn, S. K. Shenoy, and R. J. Lefkowitz, "A unique mechanism of beta-blocker action: carvedilol stimulates beta-arrestin signaling," *Proceedings of the National Academy of Sciences USA* 104, no. 42 (October 2007): 16657–62.

M. T. Drake, J. D. Violin, E. J. Whalen, J. W. Wisler, S. K. Shenoy, and R. J. Lefkowitz, "Beta-arrestin-biased agonism at the beta2-adrenergic receptor," *Journal of Biological Chemistry* 283, no. 9 (February 2008): 5669–76.

A. K. Shukla, J. D. Violin, E. J. Whalen, D. Gesty-Palmer, S. K. Shenoy, and R. J. Lefkowitz, "Distinct conformational changes in beta-arrestin report biased agonism at seven-transmembrane receptors," *Proceedings of the National Academy of Sciences USA* 105, no. 29 (July 2008): 9988–93.

7. The first papers from Brian Kobilka and colleagues reporting the crystal structure of the beta-2-adrenergic receptor are:

S. G. Rasmussen, H. J. Choi, D. M. Rosenbaum, T. S. Kobilka, F. S. Thian, P. C. Edwards, M. Burghammer, V. R. Ratnala, R. Sanishvili, R. F. Fischetti, G. F. Schertler, W. I. Weis, and B. K. Kobilka, "Crystal structure of the human beta-2 adrenergic G-protein-coupled receptor," *Nature* 450, no. 7168 (November 2007): 383–7.

D. M. Rosenbaum, V. Cherezov, M. A. Hanson, S. G. Rasmussen, F. S. Thian, T. S. Kobilka, H. J. Choi, X. J. Yao, W. I. Weis, R. C. Stevens, and B. K. Kobilka, "GPCR engineering yields high-resolution structural insights into beta2-adrenergic receptor function," *Science* 318, no. 5854 (November 2007): 1266–73.

V. Cherezov, D. M. Rosenbaum, M. A. Hanson, S. G. Rasmussen, F. S. Thian, T. S. Kobilka, H. J. Choi, P. Kuhn, W. I. Weis, B. K. Kobilka, and R. C. Stevens, "High-resolution crystal structure of an engineered human beta2-adrenergic G protein-coupled receptor," *Science* 318, no. 5854 (November 2007): 1258–65.

8. The paper from Kobilka and colleagues reporting the crystal structure of the beta-2-adrenergic receptor in complex with a G protein is:

S. G. Rasmussen, B. T. DeVree, Y. Zou, A. C. Kruse, K. Y. Chung, T. S. Kobilka, F. S. Thian, P. S. Chae, E. Pardon, D. Calinski, J. M. Mathiesen, S. T. Shah, J. A. Lyons, M. Caffrey, S. H. Gellman, J. Steyaert, G. Skiniotis, W. I. Weis, R. K. Sunahara, and B. K. Kobilka, "Crystal structure of the beta-2 adrenergic receptor-Gs protein complex," *Nature* 477, no. 7366 (July 2011): 549–55.

21. Eat More Chocolate, Win More Nobel Prizes

1. The reference for the article about the connection between chocolate consumption and Nobel Prizes is:

F. H. Messerli, "Chocolate consumption, cognitive function, and Nobel laureates," *New England Journal of Medicine* 367 (October 2012): 1562–4.

22. Nobel Week

1. A useful trick in X-ray crystallography is to generate antibodies against the target protein of interest and then use those antibodies to stabilize the protein in a particular conformation in order to obtain a better image. However, antibodies from humans (and most species) have four subunits—two heavy chains and two light chains—so they can be a bit cumbersome to use in this manner and in some cases may be too large (with a molecular weight of ~150,000 daltons) to access certain epitopes on the target protein. In contrast, antibodies from camelids (such as llamas) are completely different in structure, having only heavy chains with no light chains. Single-variable antibody domains prepared from such heavy-chain-only antibodies are much smaller than conventional antibodies (with a molecular weight ~15,000 daltons) and can thus access otherwise

cryptic epitopes on proteins. For this reason, Brian Kobilka worked with Jan Steyaert from the Vrije Universiteit Brussels in Belgium to develop some of these so-called "nanobodies" from llamas to stabilize the beta-2 adrenergic receptor in particular conformations in X-ray crystallography experiments.

2. There are many literary and cinematic representations of the Nobel Ceremony and Banquet that provide more details of these glamorous events than the thumbnail sketch provided in my account. I recommend *Reindeer with King Gustaf: What to Expect When Your Spouse Wins the Nobel Prize* by Anita Laughlin. Her husband Robert Laughlin won the Nobel Prize in Physics in 1998, and subsequently she wrote this lighthearted memoir recounting their experiences during Nobel Week. I also recommend *The Prize*, a novel by Irving Wallace, which was made into a 1963 movie starring Paul Newman. This book and movie are obviously set in an earlier era, but many of the traditions of Nobel Week are still the same. Finally, I recommend *The Wife*, an outstanding 2018 movie that contains many scenes from Nobel Week. Glenn Close was nominated for an Oscar for her work in this film.

3. The Office of the Nobel Foundation handles all of the business associated with receiving the Nobel Prize. One thing I did in this office was sign a book that has been signed by all previous Nobel Laureates. This office also deals with the various financial aspects of the prize. The size of the monetary award associated with the Nobel Prize varies from year to year, depending on the state of the Nobel endowment. In 2012, the amount of the monetary award was equivalent to $1.2 million, which in the case of the Chemistry Prize was split evenly between Brian and me. At the Office of the Nobel Foundation, I worked with the staff there to pay off the Nobel Week expenses for my family members and guests from the Nobel Prize money, such that these expenses were just subtracted and paid off before the money was wired to my bank account. Additionally, I was able to purchase several replicas of my Nobel Medal. One of these replicas is currently displayed on the Duke campus, another is at my house, and a third is in my office. The actual Nobel Medal is made of solid gold and therefore too valuable to just have laying around on my desk, so it resides in a safe deposit box.

23. The New Normal

1. Another invitation that I accepted during this period was to a Lindau Meeting. These meetings are similar to the Academy of Achievement summits in allowing students to mingle with high achievers, although the Lindau Meetings are more specifically focused on having young people from around the world interact with Nobel Laureates. The Lindau meetings have been running since 1951 as an annual series, always held in Lindau, Bavaria, Germany. I was invited each year after 2012 and was finally able to make it in 2018. I had a tremendous experience at the meeting and greatly enjoyed my interactions with all the students as well as the other Laureates from different fields.

2. Videos of my ceremonial first pitch at the Durham Bulls game can be found here:

https://www.youtube.com/watch?v=Pfq28YW5Glg
https://www.youtube.com/watch?v=PiRoICrVxKA

3. References for my lab's recent work on the structural basis of receptor interactions with beta-arrestins include:

A. K. Shukla, A. Manglik, A. C. Kruse, K. Xiao, R. I. Reis, W.-C.- Tseng, D. Staus, D. Hilger, S. Uysal, L. Y. Huang, M. Paduch, P. T. Shukla, A. Koide, S. Kide, W. I. Weis, A. A. Kossiakoff, B. K. Kobilka, and R. J. Lefkowitz, "Structure of active β-arrestin 1 bound to a G protein-coupled receptor phosphopeptide," *Nature* 497, no. 7447 (May 2013): 137–142.

A. K. Shukla, G. H. Westfield, K. Xiao, R. I. Reis, L.-Y. Huang, P. Tripathi-Shukla, J. Qian, S. Li, A. Blanc, A. N. Oleskie, A. M. Dosey, M. Su, C.-R. Liang, L.-L. Gu, J.-M. Shan, X. Chen, R. Hanna, M. Choi, X. J. Yao, B. U. Klink, A. W. Kahsai, S. S. Sidhu, S. Koide, P. A. Penczek, A. A. Kossiakoff, V. L. Woods, B. K. Kobilka, G. Skiniotis, and R. J. Lefkowitz, "Visualization of arrestin recruitment by a G-protein–coupled receptor," *Nature* 512, no. 7513 (June 2014): 218–234.

A. R. B. Thomsen, B. Louffe, T. J. Cahill, A. K. Shukla, J. T. Tarrasch, A. M. Dosey, A. W. Kahsai, R. T. Strachan, B. Pani, J. P. Mahoney, L. Huang, B. Breton, R. K. Sunahara, G. Skiniotis, M. Bouvier, and R. J. Lefkowitz, "GPCR-G Protein-β-Arrestin Super-Complex Mediates Sustained G Protein Signaling," *Cell* 166, no. 4 (August 2016): 907–919.

T. J. Cahill, A. R. B. Thomsen, J. T. Tarrasch, B. Plouffee, A. H. Nguyen, F. Yang, L.-Y. Huang, A. W. Kahsai, D. L. Bassoni, B. J. Gavino, J. E. Lamerdin, S. Triest, A. K. Shukla, B. Berger, J. Little, A. Antar, A. Blanc, C.-X. Qu, X. Chen, K. Kawakami, A. Inoue, J. Aoki, J. Steyaert, J.-P. Sun, M. Bouvier, G. Skiniotis, and R. J. Lefkowitz, "Distinct conformations of GPCR-β-arrestin complexes mediate desensitization, signaling, and endocytosis," *Proceedings of the National Academy of Sciences USA* 114, no. 10 (March 2017): 2562–2567.

A. H. Nguyen, A. R. B. Thomsen, T. J. Cahill, R. Huang, L. Y. Huang, T. Marcink, O. B. Clarke, S. Heissel, A. Masoudi, D. Ben-Hail, F. Samaan, V. P. Dandey, Y. Z. Tan, C. Hong, J. P. Mahoney, S. Triest, J. Little, X. Chen, R. Sunahara, J. Steyaert, H. Molina, Z. Yu, A. des Georges, and R. J. Lefkowitz, "Structure of an endosomal signaling GPCR-G protein-β-arrestin megacomplex," *Nature Structural and Molecular Biology* 26, no. 12 (December 2019): 1123–1131.

D. P. Staus, H. Hu, M. J. Robertson, A. L. W. Kleinhenz, L. M. Wingler, W. D. Capel, N. R. Latorraca, R. J. Lefkowitz, and G. Skiniotis, "Structure of the M2 muscarinic receptor-β-arrestin complex in a lipid nanodisc," *Nature* 579, no. 7798 (March 2020): 297–302.

24. The Art of Mentoring

1. The reference for the article in which Joe Goldstein coined the terms "PAIDS" and "technical courage" is:

J. L. Goldstein, "On the origin and prevention of PAIDS (Paralyzed Academic Investigator's Disease Syndrome)," *The Journal of Clinical Investigation* 78, no. 3 (September 1986): 848–54.

ACKNOWLEDGMENTS

My coauthor, Randy Hall, and I would like first and foremost to thank our wives. Randy's wife, Liberty, provided detailed feedback and suggested edits on early drafts of most of the chapters in this book. My wife, Lynn, also provided a number of constructive comments. We thank our wives for their help with the development of this book and also for their constant love and support.

We would like to thank various friends and colleagues who read early drafts of certain chapters and provided useful feedback: Alissa Wall Kleinhenz, Brendan Balint, TrangKimberly Nguyen, D. Scott Campbell, and Trish Ballantyne. Fact-checking of certain stories was kindly provided by Arna Brandel, Marc Caron, Brian Kobilka, Jeff Benovic, Henrik Dohlman, Jerry Olefsky, Joe Goldstein, Sven Lidin, Frank Shea, Ben Spiller, and Ralph Snyderman. Outstanding administrative assistance (past and present) was provided by Donna Addison, Joanne Bisson, Victoria Brennand, Elizabeth Hall, Mary Holben, Quivetta Lennon, Icee Li, Darby Jo Pocock, Diane Sawyer, Janet Taylor, and Julie Turnbough.

We thank our amazing agent, Jim Levine, as well as his assistant, Courtney Paganelli, and the rest of the team at Levine Greenberg Rostan Literary Agency. We also thank our exceptional editor, Jessica Case, our eagle-eyed copy editor, Peter Kranitz, and everyone at Pegasus Books.

Most importantly, major thanks and credit need to be given to all past and current members of the Lefkowitz lab, who created the Nobel-Prize-winning body of work described in this book. This incredible group of scientists includes: Seungkirl Ahn, Shahab Akhter, Wayne Alexander, Lee Allen, Jeff Arriza, Håvard Attramadal, Nick Barden, William Barnes, Jeff Benovic, Nanette Bishopric, Adi Blanc, Jeremy Blitzer, Mark Bolanowski, Michel Bouvier, Terri Brenneman, Erin Bressler, Margaret Briggs, Chad Brown, Ernst Bürgisser, Sheng Cai, Tom Cahill, Paul Campbell, Darrell Capel, Kathleen Caron, Marc Caron, Rick Cerione, Arnab Chatterjee, Minyong Chen, Jing "Ruth" Chen, Wei Chen, Yishan Cheng, Minjung Choi, Audrey Claing, William Clarke, Sheila Collins, Mei Cong, Susanna Cotecchia, Yehia Daaka, Kiefer Daniel, Laura Davidson, Albert Davies, Mardee Delahunty, André de Léan, Greg Della Rocca, Scott DeWire, Ken Dickinson, Henrik Dohlman, Matthew Drake, Mark Drazner, Sabrina Exum, Annick Fargin, David Feldman, Mark Fereshteh, Michael Field, Zoey Fredericks, Neil Freedman, Jennifer Freeman, Tom Frielle, Aditi Garikipati, Tiffany Garrison, Diane Gesty-Palmer, Larry Goldstein, Tom Gore, Randy Hall, Josh Hammer, Art Hancock, Makoto Hara, Kathryn Harley, Emily Harris, Bill Hausdorff, Brian Hawes, Jim Heinsimer, Greg Heintz, Mark Hnatowich, Brian Hoffman, Dan Houtz, Liaoyuan Hu, Dacia Hunton, Liyin Huang, Teng-Yi "Roy" Huang, Guido Iaccarino, Chris Ingersoll, Jim Inglese, Grace Irons, Xinrong Jiang, Alem Kahsai, Humphrey Kendall, Richard Kent, Khuda Dad Khan, Brian Kilpatrick, Jihee Kim, Klim King, Michael Kjelsberg, Alissa Wall Kleinhenz, Andrew Kleist, Bjoern Klink, Brian Kobilka, Tong Sun Kobilka, Wally Koch, Trudy Kohout,

Jeff Kovacs, Kathy Krueger, Hitoshi Kurose, Madan Kwatra, Chris Lam, Lucie Langevin, Tom Lavin, Ricky Lebovitz, Jungmin Mina Lee, Frederik Leeb-Lundberg, Angus Li, Steve Liggett, Lee Limbird, Fannie Lin, Yuan Lin, Mathew Lo, Martin Lohse, Jon Lomasney, Wulfing Lorenz, Lou Luttrell, Sandy Macrae, Negin Martin, Stephanie Martin, Ali Masoudi, Hiro Matsui, Stuart Maudsley, Federico Mayor, Patsy McDonald, Thomas Michel, John Mickey, Carmelo Milano, Bill Miller, Chobi Mukherjee, Debra Mullikin-Kilpatrick, Hiro Nakata, Ponnal Nambi, Canan Nebigil, Chris Nelson, Kurt Newman, Anthony Nguyen, Kelly Nobles, Lina Obeid, Brian O'Dowd, Jim Onorato, Martin Opperman, Jacek Ostrowski, Natalia Pakharukova, Biswaranjan "Bullet" Pani, Alan Payne, Sturgis Payne, Gang Pei, Karsten Peppel, Steve Perry, Kristen Pierce, Linda Pike, Julie Pitcher, Steve Plonk, Tom Povsic, Richard Premont, David Price, John Qian, Keshava Rajagopal, Sudar Rajagopal, Nadeem Rahman, Michael Raisch, Richard Randall, John Raymond, John Regan, Lindsay Rein, Rosana Reis, Eric Reiter, Xiu-Rong Ren, Kris Riebe, Michael Rockman, Neil Roth, Greg Sabo, Philippe Samama, Mika Scheinin, Doug Schocken, Deb Schwinn, Kunal Shah, Sudha Shenoy, Rob Shorr, Arun Shukla, Dave Sibley, Stella Sieber, Bob Spurney, Jeff Stadel, Dean Staus, Gary Stiles, Bob Stoffel, Carl Stone, Ryan Strachan, Cathy Strader, Ruth Strasser, Warren Strittmatter, Mark Strohsacker, Dan Stroik, Berta Strulovici, Jinpeng Sun, Yuting Tang, Rob Tate, Michael Tharp, Alex Thomsen, Akira Tohgo, Kazushige Touhara, Prachi Tripathi-Shukla, Bie Shung Tsai, Blossom Tewelde, Ron Uhing, Vivek Upadhyay, Bruno Valan, Ron Vale, Tim van Biesen, Jon Violin, Vladimir Voiekov, Rob Walters, Mei Wang-Casey, Huijin "Jack" Wei, Michael Wessels, Erin Whalen, Jarl Wikberg, Rusty Williams, Sandy Williams, Laura Wingler, Jim Wisler, Scott Witherow, Kevin Xiao, Helen Yao, Susan Yim, Taka Yoshimasa, Steven Yu, Musa Zamah, David Zang, Xingdong Zhang, Xiao Zhu, and Dave Zidar.

Thanks also to the many undergraduates, medical students, and technicians who came through the lab for short periods of time but could not be listed here due to space considerations. Additionally, thanks and deepest appreciation to the multitude of collaborators who contributed to the lab's discoveries and publications over the years. Finally, thanks to everyone in the Duke community for making Duke such a wonderful place to call home.

INDEX

A

Abboud, Francois (Frank), 86–87
Abel Award, 170
Abraham Lincoln: The War Years, 3
ACE inhibitors, 165
acromegaly, 40, 53, 113
ACTH, 43, 46–48
Addison, Donna, 122, 214
adenosine triphosphate (ATP), 49
adenylyl cyclase, 105, 125, 168
adrenaline, 56–58, 99–100, 144, 165
adrenaline receptors, 57–58, 139
adrenergic receptors, 58, 73–75,
    98–99, 131–135, 139, 174, 196. *See
    also* receptors
Aerobics, 45
Ahlquist, Raymond, 98–99
Ahn, Seungkirl, 214–215
Albert Einstein Medical Center,
    33–34, 171
aldosterone, 56
Alexander, Wayne, 74
alpha receptors, 98–99, 107. *See also*
    receptors
alpha-1 adrenergic receptor, 138–139,
    174–176
alpha-1 receptors, 107, 138–139,
    174–176

alpha-2 adrenergic receptor, 138–139
alpha-2 receptor, 138–139
alprenolol binding assay, 73–75, 100
ambulance personnel, 111
American Academy of Achievement,
    240–241
American Federation for Clinical
    Research (AFCR), 76, 78
American Heart Association, 64
American Society for Clinical Investi-
    gation (ASCI), 139–140, 182
amphibians, studies on, 100–103
anatomy class, 15, 121
Anfinsen, Christian, 56
angina, 1, 149–151
angiotensin receptor, 201
angiotensin-converting enzyme
    (ACE), 165
animals, studies on, 20, 41, 100–103,
    174–176
Anlyan, Bill, 85–86
antiwar demonstrations, 39
anxiety issues, 3, 151–152, 156
aortic stenosis, 171
aortic valve transplant, 171
Arnold, Frances, 241
arrestin, 146–147, 196, 200–202,
    248

arthritis, 21–22
"Associated Kremsdorf Descendants" (AKD), 4–5, 265
Associated Press, 167–168, 179–180
Association of American Physicians (AAP), 140, 182–185
asthma, 19
atenolol, 165
atherosclerosis, 12, 151, 162
Attramadal, Håvard, 146
auscultation, 116
awards, 169–170, 185–196, 207, 213–214, 224–225, 231–232, 241–244, 249, 267. *See also* scientific prizes
Axel, Richard, 196

B
Bader, Mortimer, 18–19, 258
Barzun, Jacques, 11
Bauer, Hank, 212
Baylor College of Medicine, 241–242
Baylor University, 83, 105, 189, 241–242
BBVA Foundation Frontiers of Knowledge Award, 191
Bell, Bill, 247
Bell, Daniel, 11–12
Benovic, Jeff, 102, 124, 127, 131, 145–146
Berra, Yogi, 212, 249
Berson, Solomon, 40
Bertin, Barbara, 267
Bertin, Mike, 267
beta adrenergic receptor kinase (BARK), 146–147
beta blockers, 57–58, 73–75, 101–103, 165, 175–176, 233
beta receptors, 57, 98–107, 115, 124–129, 132–136, 139–140, 144–147, 165, 174–176, 197. *See also* receptors

beta-1 adrenergic receptor, 137–138, 200
beta-1 receptors, 139, 142
beta-2 adrenergic receptors, 124–129, 136–139, 168, 175, 181, 196–206, 226, 260
beta-2 receptors, 138–139, 144–147, 175
beta-3 receptor, 139
beta-adrenergic receptors, 58, 73–75, 98–100, 114–115, 124, 129, 146–147, 200–201
beta-arrestins, 146–147, 196, 200–202, 248
binding assays, 48–50, 73–75, 99–101
biochemistry, 16, 51, 65–66, 103–107, 114, 224, 233
biophysics, 206, 248
Birnbaumer, Lutz, 49–50, 83–84, 105
blastomycosis, 113
bodybuilding, 8
Bouvier, Michel, 145
Brandel, Arna, 9–13, 16–17, 23, 27, 32–33, 38–39, 44–45, 51–53, 58–60, 67–69, 110–115, 131, 141–143, 148–150, 153
breathing issues, 32–34, 117, 171
Brodhead, Dick, 189
Bronx, life in, 2–11
Bronx, revisiting, 264–268
Bronx High School of Science, 7–10, 265–268
Brown, Mike, 229
Brownian motion, 147
Bruce, Lenny, 11
Buck, Linda, 196
bulimia, 35–36
Bürgisser, Ernst, 106
Burnett, Carol, 240
Bush, George W., 189–190
Bush, Laura, 190

C

cadavers, 15–16, 82

Cambridge City Hospital, 61

Cameron Indoor Stadium, 214–216, 242

cancer, 60, 159, 174, 267

car accident, 27–28, 110–112

cardiac catheterization, 150–151

cardiac disease, 162, 172, 176, 217. *See also* heart disease

cardiac health, 45–46, 149–151, 158–164

cardiac hypertrophy, 176

cardiology, 1–2, 50, 56–59, 63–64, 116, 149–151

cardiopulmonary bypass machine, 154

cardiovascular disease, 1–6, 12, 158–166. *See also* heart disease

Carey, Andy, 212

Carlsson, Arvid, 195

Carmichael, Stokely, 10

Caron, Marc, 70–71, 73–74, 96–102, 124, 127, 131, 137, 200

catheter procedure, 1–2, 151

cats, studies on, 20

cDNA libraries, 128–129

Cella, Silvio, 62–63

Centers for Disease Control, 24

Cerione, Rick, 96–97, 103–104, 151, 211, 252

Chargaff, Erwin, 16

chemical separation, 46–48

chocolate consumption, 216–218

cholesterol levels, 162–165

chronic asthma, 19

Churchill, Winston, 3, 161, 170

civil rights movement, 10

clinical conferences, 164–165

clinical work, 50, 55–56, 89, 92, 108–122

cognitive concerns, 155–157

Collins, Francis, 240

Collins, Judy, 46

Columbia University, 11–21, 24–25, 30–32, 216, 266

Columbia-Presbyterian Medical Center, 17–18, 25–30, 34–35, 38, 50, 171

"Comparison of the Theories of Class Structure of Karl Marx and Max Weber," 11

competitive instincts, 74, 84, 104–105, 131–135, 161

concentration camps, 263

Cook, Robin, 16

Cooper, Kenneth, 45–46

Cornell University, 151, 252

coronary artery disease, 151–153, 158–166. *See also* heart disease

Cosgriff, Stuart, 35–37

Cosmopolitan, 180

Cotecchia, Susanna, 107, 138–139

cough suppressants, 20

Crestor, 164

Crick, Francis, 16, 134

Curie, Marie, 169

cyanosis, 33

cyclase, 105, 125, 168

cyclic AMP levels, 49–50, 57, 105

Czestochowa, Poland, 262–265

D

Daniel, Prince, 236–237

data versus storytelling, xiv, 18–21, 258–259

Davis, Chester, 94–95

Dean, John, 68–69

"Death Project," 197–207

dementia, 159

depression, 44–46, 150, 156

dermatology team, 112–113
desensitization, 144–147
DeWire, Scott, 202
diabetes, 159
diet/nutrition, 162–164
DiMaggio, Joe, 115–116
Dixon, Richard, 125–126, 131, 137
DNA libraries, 125, 128–129
DNA sequencing, 124–128, 134–137.
    See also gene sequencing
DNA structure, 134
doctor, goal of becoming, 6, 10–20,
    23–25, 29–37, 44, 50–55
"doctor draft," 23–24
doctor-patient relationships, 20–21,
    35–37, 52–53, 116–118
Dohlman, Henrik, 127, 142, 260
Donahue, Jean, 266
Donovan, 192
double helix, 134
Double Helix, The, 134
*Dr. Dean Ornish's Program for
    Reversing Heart Disease*, 162
Duke, James B., 71
Duke University, xiii, 64–65, 70–71,
    120, 149, 213–216, 242, 247
Duke University Medical Center, 1,
    64–76, 85–89, 92, 96, 101, 104–
    106, 113–116, 120–122, 126–129,
    149, 152, 173, 178, 184–185, 189,
    211–216, 259
Durham Bulls, 245, 247
Durham Herald-Sun, 207, 211
Durham Veteran Affairs (VA) Med-
    ical Center, 115–118
Dzau, Victor, 247

E
Eastern medicine traditions, 22
eating disorders, 35–36

Einstein, Albert, 147, 169, 264
emergencies, treating, 110–112, 119–
    121. *See also* ER experiences
emergency medical technicians, 111
enalapril, 165
endocrine disorders, 40
Engel, Ms., 266–267
enzymes, 103–105, 145–146, 164–
    165, 176
epiglottitis, 33–34
epilepsy, 119–121, 199
ER experiences, 17–18, 28–29, 54–55,
    60–62
Erlenmeyer, Fritzie, 69–70
exercise regimen, 158–164. *See also*
    physical activity
exons, 129

F
family gatherings, 4–5, 265
family roots, 262–268
Fargin, Annick, 139
father-son relationship, 2–6, 12–13,
    22–23, 44–45
Fauci, Tony, 183
Federation of American Societies for
    Experimental Biology, 172
Federman, Dan, 58–59
Feibush, Joseph, 6, 8, 44
Feynman, Richard, xiii
"fight-or-flight" response, 56–57
fitness challenges, 5, 8
Flare, 180
Ford, Harrison, 245
Ford, Whitey, 212
Frankel, Gene, 8, 267
Frankfurt, Harry, 182
Fredrickson, Don, 95
Frielle, Tom, 127, 137–138, 142–144,
    260

frogs, studies on, 100–103
Frontiers of Knowledge Award, 191
fungal infection, 113

G

G proteins, 49–50, 104–105, 125,
  137–139, 146–147, 168–169, 178,
  200–206, 226
G-21 sequence, 137–139
Gabriel, Peter, 241
Gay, Bill, 94–95
Geller, Harriet Cohen, 267
gene encoding, 124–132, 136–137
gene libraries, 128–129
gene sequencing, 124–146, 197
Genentech, 125, 127, 149
Gibson, Bob, 61
Gilman, Al, 49–50, 83, 84, 104–105,
  168, 169, 207
Giuliani, Rudy, 247
glucagon binding, 49–50, 56
Golden, June, 267
Goldstein, Joe, 182–183, 229,
  254–255
Goldwater Memorial Hospital, 21,
  162
Gong Show, The, 83
Gordon, Mrs., 9–10
Gordon Research Conferences,
  81–84, 104
graduation, college, 13
graduation, high school, 10
graduation, medical school, 23–24
grand mal seizure, 119–121
Green Berets, 39
Greengard, Paul, 195
Greenwich Village, 11
grief, 45–46
growth hormone, 40, 53
GTP-sensitive factor, 49–50

guanosine triphosphate, 49–50
Gurdon, John, 209
Gustaf, King Carl XVI, 229
gym class, 5

H

Haber, Edgar, 56, 59, 64, 69–70
Halcion, 79, 80
Hall, Bill, 184
Hall, Randy, xiii, xiv
Hardman, Joel, 83
Harrison, Steve, 200, 202–203
Harvard University, 16, 30–32, 50,
  64–68, 70, 105, 197, 199–200, 202
health improvements, 45–46,
  158–164
healthy diet, 162–164
heart attacks, 2, 5–6, 9, 12, 22–23,
  44, 62, 64, 150, 267–268
heart bypass surgery, 151–159, 171
heart disease, 22–23, 45–50, 56–57,
  149–153, 158–166, 171–176, 217,
  267–268. *See also* heart issues
heart failure, 171, 176
Heart Failure Society of America, 188
Heart Institute, 47
heart issues, 1–6, 9, 12, 22–23, 116,
  149–151, 171–176
heart-lung machine, 154
Hebrew University of Jerusalem, 134
Hemingway, Ernest, 170
hemothorax, 117
Henley, Nadine, 93
high blood pressure, 159, 165
Hökfelt, Tomas, 213
Holocaust, 263, 265
Holocaust Museum, 263
Holy Grail quest, 123–136
Hong Kong Convention and Exhibi-
  tion Centre, 186–187

honorary award, 188
honorary degrees, 241–242, 244
hormone receptors, 43, 47–49, 168, 189
hormones, growth, 40, 53
Houston Texans, 242
Howard Hughes Medical Institute (HHMI), 90–97, 103, 106, 144, 256
Hughes, Howard, 91, 93–94
human genome, 134–135, 147, 204, 240
Human Genome Project, 134, 240
hypercholesterolemia, 164
hypertension, 159, 165
hypochondria, 17, 22–23, 150
hypokalemic alkalosis, 35–36, 116

I
Ignarro, Louis, 240
immune receptors, 107
insurance physicals, 60
internship experiences, 25–39
introns, 129
intubations, 54, 154–155
investigator positions, 72, 90–96, 106–109, 144, 170, 200, 254–258

J
Jagger, Mick, 190–191, 224
Jeopardy!, 177–181
jogging, 46
Johns Hopkins, 126
journalists, 179–182, 210–212, 224, 229
"junk DNA," 129. *See also* DNA

K
Kandel, Eric, 195
Karolinska Institute, 195, 235–236

kashrut, 163
Keller, Chef Thomas, 240
Kennedy, John F., 18
Kennedy, Robert, 35
kidney disease, 31–32
kinase, 145–147, 176
King, Martin Luther, Jr., 170
Kobilka, Brian, 123–132, 137–144, 203–206, 209–210, 220, 224–229, 231–235, 241, 244, 254–255, 260
Kobilka, Tong Sun, 126–127, 143, 205–206, 220, 231, 260
Koch, Wally, 176
Kong, Dave, 1–2, 151
Kovacs, Jeff, 214–215, 247
Krebs, Ed, 144–145
Kremsdorf family, 4–5, 263–265
Krzyzewski, Mike, 214–216, 242–243
Kurtz, Bob, 267

L
Late Show with David Letterman, The, 243
leadership seminars, 242
Leaf, Alex, 58–59, 67–68
Léan, André de, 105–107
lectures, 113–115, 118, 152, 182–183, 192–195, 218, 225–226. *See also* research conferences; speaking engagements
Leeb-Lundberg, Fredrik, 107
Lefkowitz, Abraham, 213
Lefkowitz, Cheryl, 32, 211
Lefkowitz, David, 23, 32–34, 62, 153, 179, 211, 241
Lefkowitz, Fannie, 213
Lefkowitz, Gary, 213
Lefkowitz, Joshua, 115, 149, 211
Lefkowitz, Larry (Noah), 23, 62
Lefkowitz, Louis, 28

Lefkowitz, Lynn, 153–157, 163, 166, 172, 177–178, 187–195, 208–210, 214–217, 220–222, 226–231, 234–241, 245, 262–265
Lefkowitz, Mara, 60, 191–192, 211, 226–228, 234, 236
Lefkowitz, Noah (Larry), 211
Lefoulon-Delalande Foundation Grand Prize for Science, 190
Leighton, Ralph, xiii
Letterman, David, 243–244
leukemia, 17
Levey, Gerald, 47
Levitzki, Alexander, 134–135
Lidin, Sven, 209
Life, 240
Limbird, Lee, 70–72, 74, 96
Lincoln, Abraham, 161
Lohse, Martin, 146
Lomasney, John, 107
lovastatin, 163
Lovejoy, Bill, 29–30, 32

M
Malcolm X, 17–18
Manger, William, 24
Mantle, Mickey, 8, 212
Marx, Karl, 11
Massachusetts General Hospital, 50–64, 66–69, 72–73, 113, 122, 159
mass-energy equivalence, 147
math, love of, 5–8
math tutor, 10
Mau, Jim, 73
McDougald, Gil, 212
McRaven, Admiral William, 240
Medal of Science, 189
media, 179–182, 210–212, 221, 224, 229, 233, 241–242

Medical College of Wisconsin, 118
medical field, love of, 15–29
medical school, 15–24
medicine, mysteries of, 15–26
mentoring others, xiv, 10, 72, 249–261
mentoring tips, 250–261
mentors, respecting, 260–261
Merck, 124–129, 131, 137
Messerli, Franz, 216, 217
Mevacor, 163
mice, studies on, 41, 174–176
Mickey, John, 121–122
midlife crisis, 148–149
Milano, Carmelo, 173–176
Mittleman, Stu, 160–161
Modrich, Paul, 242
molecular biology, 124–128, 173–174, 254
molecular cardiology, 64
moonlighting jobs, 60–63
morphine, 21, 28, 202
Morris, Jim, 150–152
Mother Teresa, 170
mother-son relationship, 3–4, 8, 170–172
Mount Sinai Hospital, 18–19, 258
Mukherjee, Chabirani "Chobi," 74
Museum of Natural History, 264
"mysteries of medicine," 15–26
"mystery physician," 110–112

N
Nambi, Ponnal, 145
narratives, xiii–xv, 18–21, 258–259
Nathans, Daniel, 126
National Academy of Sciences, 47–48, 71, 135, 205
National Institutes of Health (NIH), 24–26, 29, 32–34, 38–56, 83, 95, 105, 108, 134, 165, 182, 184, 240

National Medal of Science, 189
National Public Radio, 211
Nature, 48, 131–133, 137, 139, 181, 206
Neer, Eva, 105
nephrology, 31–32, 118
New England Journal of Medicine, 31, 216
"new normal," 239–248
New York City, life in, 2–11, 15–17
New York City, revisiting, 264–268
New York Times, 3, 172, 210
New York University, 14
New York Yankees, 7–8, 115, 212, 245–249
Newman, Kurt, 121–122
NIH Clinical Center, 40–41
Nixon, Richard, 69
Nobel, Alfred, 218
Nobel Banquet, 219, 227–230, 235–236
Nobel Ceremony, 227–230
Nobel Committee, 16, 196, 206–210, 222, 224, 244
Nobel Foundation, 168, 223, 231, 235–236
Nobel Lecture, 218, 225–226
Nobel Medal, 229, 235
Nobel Monument, 264–265
Nobel Museum, 223–224
Nobel Prize, xiii, 16, 49–50, 134, 144–145, 167–176, 195–196, 207–249, 264–266
Nobel Symposium, 195–196, 206, 229
Nobel Week, 220–238
noradrenaline, 57–58, 73–75, 195
norepinephrine, 195
Normark, Staffan, 208–210
nuclear hormone receptors, 189
nucleotide triphosphates, 49

O

Obama, Barack, 189, 220–221, 242–243
Obama, Michelle, 221
odds, surviving against, 158–166
odorant receptors, 178–181, 196
Olefsky, Jerry, 80
Olympics, 184, 214
O'Malley, Bert, 189
On Bullshit, 182
opiates, 21, 28, 30, 155, 202, 233
Ornish, Dean, 162–163
O'Shea, Erin, 94
oxytocin receptor, 114–115

P

pain relief, 22, 28–29
paparazzi, 222–224, 229
"Paralyzed Academic Investigator's Disease Syndrome" (PAIDS), 254
paregoric, 30
Pares, Serge, 199
Pastan, Ira, 43, 56, 83, 253–254
patient histories, 116–118
patient-doctor relationships, 20–21, 35–37, 52–53, 116–118
Pauling, Linus, 134
peptide hormone, 48
phosphorylation, 145–147, 176
photoelectric effect, 147
physical activity, 1–2, 45–46, 158–164
physicals, 60
physician-patient, xv
physician-scientist, xv, 108–109
pituitary hormones, 53
placebo effect, 21–22, 30
Poitier, Sydney, 240
Poland, visiting, 262–264
Polish Academy of Sciences, 262

prison doctors, 24

Proceedings of the National Academy of Sciences (PNAS), 48

protein phosphorylation, 145–147, 176

Public Health Service, 24, 39, 108, 184

public speaking, 48, 75. *See also* speaking engagements

publishing experiences, 47–48, 103, 131–132, 204

pulmonary fibrosis, 18–19, 171

purified receptors, 99–105, 124–127, 138–139, 168, 197

R

radioactive beta blockers, 73–75, 101–102

radioactive binding assay, 73–75, 99–101

radioactive iodine, 49

radioactive ligands, 73, 128

radioactive noradrenaline binding, 73–75

radioactive tritium, 73–74

radioimmunoassay, 40, 48

radiolabeling, 48, 73–74, 145

radioligand binding assays, 73–75

"radioreceptor assay," 48

Rall, Ed, 48

Raymond, John, 118, 139, 169

receptors

    adrenaline, 57–58, 139

    adrenergic, 58, 73–75, 98–99, 131–135, 139, 174, 196

    alpha, 98–99, 107

    alpha-1, 107, 138–139, 174–176

    alpha-1 adrenergic, 138–139, 174–176

    alpha-2, 138–139

    alpha-2 adrenergic, 138–139

angiotensin, 201

    beta, 57, 98–107, 115, 124–129, 132–136, 139–140, 144–147, 165, 174–176, 197

    beta-1, 139, 142

    beta-1 adrenergic, 137–138, 200

    beta-2, 138–139, 144–147, 175

    beta-2 adrenergic, 124–129, 136–139, 168, 175, 181, 196–206, 226, 260

    beta-3, 139

    beta-adrenergic, 58, 73–75, 98–100, 114–115, 124, 129, 146–147, 200–201

    existence of, 98–107

    hormone, 43, 47–49, 168, 189

    immune, 107

    nuclear hormone receptors, 189

    odorant receptors, 178–181, 196

    oxytocin, 114–115

    purified, 99–105, 124–127, 138–139, 168, 197

    scrotonin, 139

    structure of, 74, 196, 197, 255

Regan, John, 107, 138

Regeneron Pharmaceuticals, 266

research conferences, 74–75, 81–84, 98–99, 104, 192–193, 239–241, 244, 257–261. *See also* research seminars; scientific meetings

research experiences, 19–20, 24–25, 32, 38–51, 55–59, 63–64, 73–75, 85–89

research seminars, 64–65, 86, 113–114, 151, 195, 247–248. *See also* research conferences

resuscitation, 54–55, 63–64

Reves, Jerry, 152, 154

Reynolds, Brian Blaine, 240

rheumatoid arthritis, 21–22

rhodopsin, 136–137, 146–147, 168, 255

Rizzuto, Phil, 212

Robertson, Gary, 42

Robison, Al, 83

Roche, 20

Rockman, Howard, 174–175

Rodbell, Marty, 48–50, 83, 168

Rolling Stones, 190, 224

Roosevelt, Theodore, 264

roots, 262–268

Rosetta Stone, 136–147, 196

Ross, Diana, 240

Ross, Elliott, 105, 125, 127–129, 131–134

Ross, John, 174

rosuvastatin, 164

Roth, Alvin, 221

Roth, Jesse, 25–26, 32, 40–43, 47–50, 56, 83, 253–254, 261

Royal Palace, 236

Royal Swedish Academy of Sciences, 208–209, 213, 222–225, 231

Rudolph, Steve, 8, 9

S

Sabiston, David, 152, 173

Sahl, Mort, 11

San Francisco Chronicle, 179

Sandburg, Carl, 3

Sanders, Charlie, 50–51

saying no, 85–89

Schindler, Oskar, 263

Schindler's List, 263

Science, 48, 204

science, love of, 7–8

science writers' conferences, 178–180

scientific meetings, 78–84, 98–99, 106, 118, 195, 235, 239–240, 251, 257–261. *See also* research conferences

scientific prizes, 170, 186–196. *See also specific prizes*

Scolnick, Ed, 124, 126

Second World War, The, 3

See, Andrew, 247

seizure, 119–121

serotonin receptors, 139

Shannon, James, 48

Shapley, Lloyd, 221

Shaw, Run Run, 186–187

Shaw Prize, 186–189, 196

Shorr, Rob, 102

Sibley, David, 145

Sigal, Irving, 126, 131

Sigler, Paul, 199

Silverman, Norm, 160–161

Simpson, O. J., 156

skills, developing, 5–8

skin lesions, 112–113

Skiniotis, Yiorgo, 206, 235

Skowron, Moose, 212

SmithKline, 79

Snyderman, Ralph, 107–108, 149, 153–155, 159–161, 211

Southwestern Medical School, 104, 125

Souza, Pete, 221

Spanish National Research Council, 191

speaking engagements, 48, 75, 84, 86, 98–99, 113–115, 118, 152, 179, 182–183, 195, 237, 240, 248, 262. *See also* lectures; research conferences

special relativity, 147

sperm research, 178–181

Spiller, Ben, 199–200, 202–203

sports team doctor, 61–62

St. Jude's Hospital, 198
Stadel, Jeff, 145
Stanford University, 203, 255
statins, 163–165
Steinbeck, John, 264
stem cell research, 209
sternotomy, 155
steroid hormone, 56
Stevens, Ray, 203–204
Sting, 241
Stockholm University, 225
Stockholm visits, 194–196, 206–249
storytelling, xiii–xv, 18–21, 116–118,
    258–259
Strader, Cathy, 124, 131, 137
stress response, 43, 53, 181–182
Strulovici, Berta, 104, 145
sub-internship experience, 20–22,
    162
Sunahara, Roger, 206, 226, 235
surgery experiences, 20–21, 41–42.
    See also heart bypass surgery
Sutherland, Earl, 83
Swedish Academy of Sciences, 208–
    209, 213, 222–225, 231

T
"Tale of Two Callings," xv
teaching experiences, 120–121. *See
    also* mentoring others
terrorist events, 198, 246–247
Thier, Sam, 30–32
Thorn, George, 93–94
Tilley, Lynn, 153
travel experiences, 76–84, 186–196,
    262–268
Trevena, 201–202
Trilling, Lionel, 11
tuberculosis, 15–16
tutoring students, 10

U
Ullrich, Axel, 125, 127–129, 131, 134
United States Public Health Service
    (USPHS), 24
University of California San Diego,
    80, 174
University of California San Fran-
    cisco, 71, 125, 253
University of Illinois, 203
University of Iowa, 86–87
University of Jerusalem, 134
University of Miami, 70
University of North Carolina, 70,
    142, 153
University of Texas Southwestern
    Medical School, 104, 125
Uppsala University, 236, 237

V
Van Trigt, Peter, 152
Vanderbilt University, 71, 96
Varmus, Harold, 16, 39, 45
Vassart, Gilbert, 180, 181
Venter, J. Craig, 134–135
ventricular fibrillation, 54–55
Victoria, Crown Princess, 236
Vietnam War, 23–26, 29, 32, 39, 44,
    108, 184
Violin, Jonathan, 202
virus research, 138, 198
von Euler, Ulf, 195
von Heijne, Gunnar, 206

W
Wallace, Andy, 64–67, 70
Washington Post, 211
Watergate hearings, 68–69
Watson, James, 16, 134
Watt, J. J., 242
Weber, Max, 11

weightlifting, 8
Whalen, Erin, 202
Wiley, Don, 197–200
Wilkins, Maurice, 16
Williams, Rusty, 70–72, 74, 125,
    127–128
Wineland, David, 221
Woodling, Gene, 212
workshops, 92–95, 107, 144
Wright, Kenny, 93, 96
Wyngaarden, Jim, 65–66, 73, 87,
    90–92

X
Xanax, 155
X-ray crystallography research, 197–
    203, 255

Y
Yale University, 29, 71–72, 199,
    236
Yalow, Rosalyn, 40
Yamanaka, Chika, 230
Yamanaka, Shinya, 209, 224, 229,
    230
Yancopoulos, George, 266
Yankee Stadium, 7–8, 245. *See also*
    New York Yankees
Yellow Berets, 38–51, 83, 108, 149,
    182–183, 229, 254